The Clinician's Guide to Chronic Disease Management for Long-Term Conditions

A cognitive–behavioural approach

Gill Furze, Jenny Donnison
and Robert JP Lewin

D0273449

The Clinician's Guide to
Chronic Disease Management for Long-Term Conditions
A cognitive–behavioural approach
Gill Furze, Jenny Donnison and Robert JP Lewin

ISBN: 978-1-905539-15-4

First published 2008

British Library Catalogue in Publication Data
A catalogue record for this book is available from the British Library

Notice
Clinical practice and medical knowledge constantly evolve. Standard safety precautions must be followed, but, as knowledge is broadened by research, changes in practice, treatment and drug therapy may become necessary or appropriate. Readers must check the most current product information provided by the manufacturer of each drug to be administered and verify the dosages and correct administration, as well as contraindications. It is the responsibility of the practitioner, utilising the experience and knowledge of the patient, to determine dosages and the best treatment for each individual patient. Any brands mentioned in this book are as examples only and are not endorsed by the Publisher. Neither the publisher nor the authors assume any liability for any injury and/or damage to persons or property arising from this publication.

The Publisher
To contact M&K Publishing write to:
M&K Update Ltd · The Old Bakery · St. John's Street
Keswick · Cumbria CA12 5AS
Tel: 01768 773030 · Fax: 01768 781099
publishing@mkupdate.co.uk
www.mkupdate.co.uk

Designed & typeset by Mary Blood
Printed in England by Reeds Printers, Penrith

Contents

List of figures

List of tables

About the authors

Gill Furze is a nurse who practised for many years in medical rehabilitation and cardiac care and prevention, and is currently Senior Research Fellow at the British Heart Foundation Care and Education Research Group at the University of York. She has co-authored (with Bob Lewin) cognitive–behavioural self-management programmes for people with heart disease (the Angina Plan, the Angioplasty Plan) and developed and continues to run the training for these. In the last 4 years more than 800 NHS staff have been trained, who have delivered these programmes to around 20,000 patients.

Bob Lewin was a social worker but retrained as a clinical psychologist and worked for many years in NHS hospitals with people with chronic illness. He pioneered the use of cognitive–behavioural self-management programmes in cardiac illness more than 20 years ago, developing and evaluating *The Heart Manual*, a programme now in use in many settings in the UK and overseas. He is currently Professor of Rehabilitation at the University of York and Director of the British Heart Foundation Care & Education Research Group. In his academic role he has conducted more than 30 research projects and published widely on managing chronic illnesses.

Jenny Donnison is a clinical psychologist with an interest in cognitive therapy. Since qualifying, Jenny has worked in Tower Hamlets, London, and in Sheffield, providing psychological therapy for adults with mental health problems, principally in primary care settings. Jenny has also maintained an interest in health psychology and the impact of chronic health problems on psychological well-being, for example through involvement in projects on coronary heart disease, asthma and diabetes.

Acknowledgements

Thanks to Sue Martindale, Moira Leahy, Jayne Levell and Linda Wilkinson for reading and commenting on chapters within the book.

Introduction

This book has been written with clinicians in mind who are caring for people with long-term or chronic conditions. Throughout the book we will refer to people with long-term conditions (rather than people with chronic disease) as our focus extends beyond disease management. We aim to provide an informative and useful resource to help clinicians understand how people deal with, and adjust to, life with a long-term condition.

The purpose therefore is not to provide the reader with an in-depth knowledge of psychological theory but instead to provide background knowledge and theory about cognitive–behavioural therapy (CBT) to develop an understanding of how people deal with and adjust to living with a long-term condition. This includes:

- exploring the concepts 'disability' and 'impairment', what the differences are and why they are important
- looking at the biomedical versus the biopsychosocial model; while these concepts have been explored elsewhere, this book gives readers the opportunity to consider what 'doing it the biopsychosocial way' means for clinicians, patients and carers
- considering beliefs about long-term conditions and why, as a clinician, it is important to understand these.

This book also provides some practical, proven resources that clinicians can use in their work supporting people with long-term conditions. These focus on tools and skills that clinicians can easily use in their everyday practice, with the aim of helping people become 'self-managers'. The tools and skills are based on cognitive–behavioural techniques, widely acknowledged as effective methods for empowering people to self-manage.

Using the book

Throughout the book theoretical concepts are illustrated by practical examples and fictitious 'case studies', demonstrating how the theory relates to practice and how it might apply to individual patients, relatives or carers. At the end of each chapter we have included a series of 'points for reflection'. These are areas you may want to consider when relating the content of this book back to your clinical practice.

Chronic disease management for long-term conditions

We hope that you enjoy the book. If you have any comments or suggestions for topics that could be included in future editions please get in touch.

Gill Furze, Jenny Donnison and Bob Lewin

Address for correspondence: Dr Gill Furze, Department of Health Science, Area 2 SRB, University of York, York, YO10 5DD UK.

Chapter 1
Cognitive–behavioural therapy

Introduction

The first part of this chapter summarises the main principles of CBT and illustrates these using fictitious case material. We then explore how CBT principles may be applied to the management of long-term conditions.

Please note: While cognitive–behavioural psychotherapy should not be undertaken without training on an accredited CBT course and appropriate clinical supervision, many of the CBT principles and techniques described may be incorporated into work with people with long-term conditions. Examples include establishing a good therapeutic relationship, working collaboratively, setting goals jointly with clients and using diaries. It is also important to ensure that any unexplained physical symptoms are assessed by the patient's primary-care physician prior to commencing psychologically informed work.

The principles of cognitive–behavioural therapy

Principles of CBT

The essentials of cognitive–behavioural therapy can be simply stated: CBT is a psychotherapeutic model, the central tenet of which is that the way we think (cognition) influences our emotions and behaviour; in turn, our behaviour and emotions influence our thinking. A central task for cognitive–behavioural psychotherapists is to enable clients to develop a deeper awareness of their thoughts and how these affect emotions (including associated physiological feelings) and behaviour. Clients are helped to explore the usefulness and validity of habitual ways of thinking and to develop new perspectives. The therapist assists clients to consider how this new perspective might be translated into making changes. Changes in behaviour can, in turn, alter thinking. In essence CBT is concerned with uncovering and exploring meaning.

CBT was developed by A.T. Beck in the 1960s. Beck was a psychoanalytically trained psychiatrist. However as he worked with depressed patients he observed that their thoughts about themselves, the world and the future were predominantly negative. He reasoned that this negatively biased and distorted thinking might be significant in the maintenance of depression (Beck, 1976). Helping patients become more aware of these negative thoughts and assisting them to develop more balanced and less catastrophic views was helpful in creating hope, alleviating low mood and changing behaviour.

Although Beck can be regarded as the originator of CBT as it is currently practiced, several psychologists prior to Beck influenced its development. The behavioural element of CBT has its origins in the work of behaviourists, notably Pavlov and Skinner. These psychologists focused their attention on observable behaviour rather than the private world of thought and emotion. From the 1950s onwards behavioural principles were applied to the alleviation of psychological problems. As behaviour therapy developed, cognitive elements were integrated, enhancing the depth and effectiveness of therapy by uncovering the idiosyncratic meaning of difficulties. For a summary of the development of CBT, see Wright *et al.* (2006).

Since Beck's early work on depression there has been a rapid expansion of CBT. CBT principles have been applied to many problems, including anxiety disorders (for example panic attacks, social anxiety and health anxiety), eating disorders (anorexia and bulimia nervosa) and post-traumatic stress disorder (PTSD). CBT has also been applied to psychosis, for example, bipolar disorder (manic depression). Additionally, work is underway to develop CBT approaches to personality disorders. The effectiveness of CBT has been supported by empirical studies (see Butler and Beck, 2000).

CBT has experienced a rapid expansion, and while it should not be regarded as a panacea, it has empirical support and is endorsed in the guidelines of the National Institute for Health and Clinical Excellence, for example, for depression and anxiety (NICE, 2004a, 2004b). Although the science underpinning CBT is sophisticated, a great strength is that CBT principles can be simply stated in ordinary language. The central ideas, that thoughts and beliefs – our individual 'take' on life – shape emotions and behaviour, has the feel of common sense. Moreover these ideas are not new. For example the Greek philosopher Epictetus (c. 55–135 AD) wrote that 'we are moved not by the things themselves but by the meanings we give them'.

Levels of cognition

Levels of cognition

As noted above, CBT is based on the idea that cognition plays a significant role in emotional difficulties and emotional well being. In CBT three levels of cognition are usually described: core beliefs or schemas, rules or assumptions, and automatic thoughts.

Core beliefs

These are the ideas that we hold about ourselves, the wider world, other people and so on. They are absolute and unconditional and may be positive or negative, for example 'I am a failure', 'I am lovable'. Core beliefs are considered to be the least accessible level of cognition and are often implicit; that is, we behave as if they are true without necessarily articulating them. Such beliefs develop as we grow up and depend on our experiences. For example a child who experienced rejection may form the belief that he or she is unlovable; a child who has experienced hurt may believe that others can't be trusted. Someone who grew up in a family where physical fitness was valued and physical vulnerability disparaged may develop the belief that physical illness equates with weakness. If such an individual falls ill, such beliefs may hasten – or hamper – their recovery. Further information about core beliefs can be found in CBT texts, for example Greenberger and Padesky (1995), Padesky and Greenberger (1995) and Wright *et al.* (2006). For further discussion of the role of beliefs in managing long-term conditions, see Chapter 3.

Assumptions or rules

Rules or assumptions are generally more accessible than core beliefs. They guide behaviour and are conditional; for example, they are often in the form of 'if...then' statements, such as 'If I work hard then I will succeed' or 'If I am rejected then I am unlovable'. Rules can also take the form of statements including unhelpfully inflexible words such as 'must', 'should', 'always' or 'never'. For example 'I must do things perfectly otherwise I am a failure'. Such rules or assumptions are helpful if realistic – for example 'I don't have to be perfect to be accepted by others'. Assisting clients to be more aware of the rules or assumptions they routinely take for granted can be useful. Clients may then consider whether such assumptions are reasonable (for example exploring the pros and cons of perfectionism) and might be helped to construct more realistic guidelines. The next step is to consider what living with the new rule might mean in practice. For example, the implications of the rule 'I must do things perfectly otherwise I am a failure' are very different from the gentler rule 'I don't have to be perfect to be accepted by others'.

Automatic thoughts and images

Most accessible are automatic thoughts and images. Such thoughts occur thousands of times each day and are fleeting. We may not be particularly aware of them but they can influence mood. Anxious people may have automatic thoughts related to imminent or future harm while depressed individuals might have thoughts related to loss. CBT assists clients to notice and challenge any unhelpful thoughts that precede, accompany and follow changes in mood and to explore relationships between thoughts, emotions, physiology and behaviour.

When working with people, particularly those struggling with disadvantage, it is important to recognise the difference between facts ('I am about to be made redundant') and automatic thoughts which may be distorted or biased ('I'll never get another job'). Depressed or anxious individuals faced with adversity may underestimate their capacity to cope, or blame themselves erroneously for their predicament. For example, a woman with low self-esteem subjected to domestic violence might attribute responsibility to herself for her partner's unacceptable behaviour. She might perhaps think 'It's my fault he's like this', leading to guilt and depression. Identifying, exploring and challenging such unhelpful attributions is appropriate. However it is important that facts are not mistaken for, or treated as, negative thoughts. If an individual faces a pressing problem such as redundancy, racism, marital separation or a failed exam it may be most productive to assist them to address the difficulty. This can be done collaboratively, for example using problem-solving strategies (see Chapter 6; Butler and Hope, 2007; Powell, 2000) or by facilitating access to appropriate agencies. For further discussion of these and related issues see Moorey (1996) and Hagan and Donnison (1999).

Case example 1

Michael, with asthma and anxiety

Michael, a first-year university student with asthma was hospitalised after experiencing severe breathing difficulties while out. The doctor in emergency thought it possible that Michael's symptoms were exacerbated by anxiety. On discharge, Michael saw his doctor and admitted that this was not the first time he had had such difficulties. His doctor suggested he talked through his asthma management with a CBT-trained specialist asthma nurse, Kath. Michael told Kath what happened. He was out with some new friends and his new girlfriend, Karen, and realised that he was becoming wheezy. He delayed using his inhaler and felt increasingly anxious. A friend called for an ambulance as Michael seemed to be fighting for breath. In the discussion that ensued, Kath asked Michael questions to elicit his thoughts, emotions, physical feelings and behaviour during the incident. His automatic thoughts and images are in bold print.

Kath: What was going through your mind as you started to notice the wheeziness?
Michael: I remember thinking '**Oh no, not again**'. And then I thought '**I don't want to use my inhaler in front of everyone**'. I hadn't told my friends or Karen about my asthma. I thought '**She'll think I'm pathetic**'.
Kath: How did you feel?
Michael: Really self-conscious and worried. I was getting breathless but I didn't want them to see me with my inhaler and make a big fuss. I get really embarrassed if people see me using the inhaler.
Kath: So you were worried people would make a fuss. I wonder what 'making a fuss' means to you?
Michael: Well I just had **this image of myself getting out my inhaler and using it and my friends saying 'What's that?' and me having to explain but being too breathless to talk**

properly and, I don't know, either them panicking or something... or maybe laughing at me... and people looking at me and maybe coming up and saying 'Are you all right?'. I hate being the centre of attention like that – I tried to hide what was happening.

Kath: It sounds like you have an image of yourself being the focus of a lot of unwanted attention. Did you notice anything happening to your body?

Michael: Well yes. The breathlessness was getting worse and I noticed my heart beating faster and I was sweating. I was feeling really anxious.

Kath: What was going through your mind as you became more anxious?

Michael: Two main things. I thought **'Oh, no! I've left it too late to use the inhaler'** and [*looks rueful*] – this is going to sound silly – but I thought **'My friends won't want to be seen with me after this.'** I suppose I started to panic.

Michael and Kath then pieced together how Michael's thoughts may have contributed to the asthma attack becoming uncontrolled (see 'Formulation' on p. 10).

A sound therapeutic relationship

Therapeutic relationships

Like all psychotherapies, the foundation of CBT is a good therapeutic alliance. Effective therapy requires a trusting relationship. Without this, people will be unwilling to discuss their difficulties. An essential part of establishing trust is practising to high ethical standards. For example, being clear at the outset about the limits of confidentiality; giving information about your role (and its limitations, such as constraints regarding the number of sessions you can offer); ensuring that you have informed consent for the work you are undertaking so that, for example, you do not drift into sensitive or distressing areas, without some discussion of what this might mean for the client. It is also essential to work within the limits of competence.

The core qualities of an effective person-centred counsellor are:

- genuineness (a capacity to be oneself or authentic with a client, while retaining boundaries appropriate to a professional helping relationship)

- unconditional positive regard and a non-judgemental stance
- an ability to experience and convey empathy (see Mearns & Thorne 1992 for a discussion of the principles and practice of person-centred counselling).

These skills can be learned and are addressed in psychotherapy or counselling training. For example empathy is demonstrated by skills such as 'active listening' in which the therapist learns to hear not only factual content but unspoken emotional nuance. The therapist learns to reflect this accurately back to clients. In this way clients both feel understood and may deepen their own understanding.

These are characteristics essential to all good therapy. It is a myth that CBT neglects the therapeutic relationship (for an account of this and other CBT myths, see Gilbert, 2006). Arguably, CBT is particularly conducive to a good alliance as it is characterised by an explicitly collaborative stance. Therapist and client work together as a team in which the client's experience, knowledge and self-knowledge are respected while the therapist contributes specific skills and expertise about CBT. In practical terms, collaboration is facilitated by helping the client set realistic goals and by jointly planning sessions. Sessions are guided by a jointly negotiated written agenda. Clients are invited to contribute to agenda-setting, ensuring that important issues are not overlooked. Prioritisation of agenda items is also done jointly. The CB therapist also explicitly invites feedback from clients, particularly discussion of anything that might result in misunderstanding or mistrust. For further discussion of the therapeutic relationship within CBT see Wright *et al.* (2006), Safran and Segal (1996) and Waddington (2002).

Guided discovery

Guided discovery

A key skill in CBT is guided discovery. This means that rather than therapists instructing or advising clients, clients are helped to discover things for themselves. Therapist and client work together like scientists to observe and record information about problems, to develop and test hypotheses about factors underpinning and maintaining difficulties, and to test these hypotheses through carefully planned tasks within and between sessions using various methods, e.g. behavioural experiments. For example, where unhelpful thoughts are identified, the therapist assists the client to explore the evidence both for and against a particular idea. Such learning is powerful and memorable and more likely to be 'owned' and accepted by the client.

A key method in guided discovery is Socratic questioning. The therapist asks a series of questions through which the client is helped to become more aware of, for example, their cognitions and how these impact on emotions and behaviour. Effective Socratic dialogue involves the therapist asking questions which the client has the knowledge to answer, for example by encouraging their reflection on previous experience. Moreover this new information will serve to inform and clarify the client's situation and facilitate increased insight and understanding. Further, good Socratic questions are prompted by the therapist's genuine curiosity rather than preconceived ideas. In this way new and surprising information may emerge involving genuine discovery. For an account of the principles of guided discovery, see Padesky (1993) and Kennerley (2007). Kath in Case example 1 uses Socratic questioning to deepen her and Michael's understanding of a key event.

Formulation (or case conceptualisation)

Formulation

CBT is guided by a formulation or case conceptualisation, developed collaboratively with clients. The formulation provides a 'road-map' to ensure the therapy has shape, direction and structure. There are several formats available for developing and presenting clinical formulations and these can be found in cognitive therapy texts. The most usual format tells the story of how problems develop, including vulnerability factors (early experiences, unhelpful beliefs and assumptions), the critical event or events that triggered the problem and which activated unhelpful beliefs and one or more examples of the presenting problem, including key maintaining factors. Information about formulation in CBT can be found in a range of CBT texts including Persons (1989) and Wright et al. (2006).

Cognitive–behavioural therapy

It is also useful to be familiar with the various models, for example those of depression (e.g. Beck *et al.*, 1979), panic disorder or social phobia (e.g. Wells, 1997) which have been developed through research. These are valuable templates onto which an individual client's unique presentation can be mapped. These models usually take the form of 'vicious cycles'; understanding these and seeing how cycles might be broken or exited can be a powerful clinical tool.

A central task of early sessions is to introduce the CBT model. This is best accomplished by taking a specific recent example of the presenting problem and exploring the sequence of thoughts, emotions, physical changes and behaviour that occurred (see Padesky & Mooney, 1990). A recent, memorable occasion when the client experienced high affect (sadness, fear, anxiety, guilt and so forth) is most useful. For further information see Greenberger and Padesky (1995), Wright *et al.* (2006) and Williams (2001).

Figure 1.1   **Emotions, thoughts and behaviours behind a patient's presenting problem**

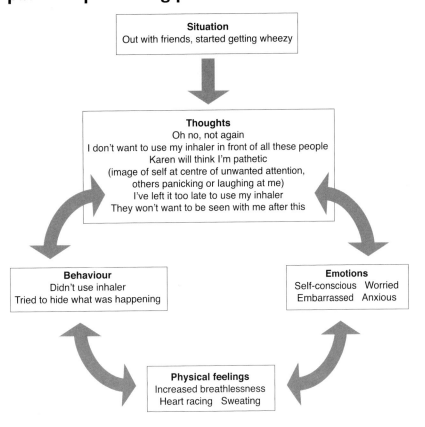

As Kath and Michael worked together to unpick the sequence of events leading to his visit to the emergency department, Kath carefully wrote down what Michael said, using a framework that linked situation, thoughts, emotions, behaviour and physical reactions. Several formats are available to guide this exercise (see Greenberger and Padesky, 1995; Williams, 2001 and Wright *et al.*, 2006).

This process enabled them to discover that Michael's self-consciousness about using his inhaler in front of others led to avoidance, resulting in an uncontrolled asthma episode. In addition it seemed possible that anxiety symptoms were exacerbating the asthma attack.

Initially CBT focuses on 'here and now' issues. In Michael's case Figure 1.1 shows the sequence of thoughts, emotions, physical sensations and behaviour maintaining the problem. Michael was able to see that his thoughts about how others might perceive him both increased his anxiety and also led him to avoid taking appropriate steps to manage the asthma attack. Developing a 'vicious cycle' formulation that describes how problems are maintained is useful because it clarifies possible points of intervention.

How did Michael's problems develop?

Although much of the work in CBT is focused on addressing difficulties in the here and now, cognitive–behavioural therapists also take account of factors leading to the problem's development. During assessment, information is collected about the client's history which will be useful in developing hypotheses about the origins of presenting problems.

In an earlier assessment session Kath had asked Michael about his history, in particular his experience of asthma. Michael described his family in positive terms. He was the youngest of two children. His parents were 'outdoor types' and Michael recalled his mother having a 'fairly robust attitude to illness'. Michael remembers being wrapped up well and sent to school even if he felt ill. He recalled two occasions at primary school when he was too poorly to stay at school and his mother was asked to collect him. He remembers feeling very miserable at these times, as if he had done something wrong. On one occasion his mother became cross when he cried, and told him 'You're pathetic'. Although he rationalised this by saying his mother was probably having a 'bad day' he became quite emotional when describing it. Michael's asthma was diagnosed when he was eleven, during the year that he made the transition to secondary school. Michael recalled that his parents played down his asthma. He remembered a time at secondary school, when he was about thirteen, when he had been teased by some older pupils for using his inhaler. He had felt humiliated; the asthma attack had been severe and he had to be taken to the school nurse. After this Michael had tried to avoid using his inhaler in public, and when he did, he often used it ineffectively in an attempt to be discreet. It transpired that there had been other occasions when his self-consciousness had compromised self-care.

Kath and Michael developed the following formulation together. Michael's early experience was of a generally happy childhood, although his Mum had a 'robust' attitude to illness and Michael recalled being sent to school when unwell. On two occasions he had to be sent home and felt bad and guilty on these occasions. He particularly recalled his mother saying that he was 'pathetic' and this appeared to be a core belief relevant to his presenting difficulties. Michael developed asthma when he was eleven and became self-conscious about his inhaler. He developed assumptions or rules relevant to his asthma management, such as 'If you ignore illness it will go away' and 'If I am ill or vulnerable I may be criticised or hurt.' A key event occurred when he was thirteen, when he was teased by older pupils about using his inhaler. This activated and reinforced his beliefs and assumptions about himself (e.g. 'I'm pathetic'), and about illness and the perceived perils of showing vulnerability (e.g. 'If I am ill or vulnerable I may be criticised or hurt').

The specific presenting problem (Figure 1.1, above) was then re-examined and Michael began to see how his childhood and teenage experiences had shaped his current difficulties.

Between-session tasks (homework)

Homework

Consistent with the use of guided discovery, CBT is an active therapy. Clients are encouraged to undertake various tasks or activities between sessions. The nature of these activities follows logically from the formulation. A common early task is to keep a diary recording key features of a problem. For example a depressed person might be encouraged to keep a diary charting their activity and fluctuations in mood over several days. An example of this type of diary can be found in Greenberger & Padesky (1995). A person experiencing panic attacks might record the frequency and severity of panic episodes, together with details on preceding and accompanying thoughts, the situations in which they occur and so on. A person with type 2 diabetes might be encouraged to keep a food diary over the course of a week to facilitate discussion about adjustments to their diet.

Kath and Michael together constructed a diary (Figure 1.2) to capture key elements of Michael's problem. After discussing the incident leading to Michael's admission they agreed it would be helpful to discover more about those times when Michael became wheezy.

Figure 1.2   Michael's asthma diary

Brief description of situation (i.e. when, where, with whom, etc.)	Emotions (0–10)	Thoughts	Physical sensations	Severity (0–10)	Outcome – what happened?
Monday 1/11, 8.30 In my room in hall of residence, alone. Started to feel wheezy	Annoyed, 2	I'll be late	Wheezy	3	Used inhaler, felt better quite quickly. Finished getting ready
Monday, 10.00 In lecture	Anxious and Embarrassed	Everyone will notice. They'll make a fuss. Will lecturer ask me if I'm OK? Should I leave now?	Wheezy, heart racing, sweating	8	Left lecture. Felt embarrassed. Used inhaler outside. Wheeziness subsided but felt anxious and upset. Didn't go back in

This type of information is helpful for several reasons. Firstly, it provides a baseline against which changes in the frequency and intensity of target problems can be measured. Secondly, it delivers valuable, specific information about the problem which feeds into the formulation, suggesting areas for change. Finally, it helps the client and therapist to record what happens when changes are made.

Cognitive–behavioural therapy

A commonly used diary in CBT is the thought record. Several formats are available (e.g. Greenberger and Padesky, 1995). The rationale for keeping a thought record flows from the CBT model – in essence fleeting and automatic thoughts can influence mood and behaviour; writing these down can allow their validity to be evaluated, facilitating development of more balanced alternatives. Where a number of thoughts occur it is useful to pinpoint the one which is most emotionally charged. Greenberger and Padesky (1995) term this the 'hot thought'. It is important to work through one or more thought records with clients to illustrate and build confidence in the method. In Case example 1 Michael identified upsetting thoughts about how others might react if he was seen using his inhaler. By using a thought record to examine evidence for and against this thought, Michael was able to see that his main evidence for thinking that he might be ridiculed or given unwelcome attention was historical, based on his schoolboy experience of being teased for using an inhaler. He also saw that his mother's response to illness had contributed to his feelings of shame about allowing others to see his physical vulnerability. Kath asked Michael if he could remember how his friends and Karen had actually responded to the asthma episode. He couldn't remember much but thought they'd been quite calm. On reflection Michael realised that his new friends and Karen had been kind and concerned after his admission and had not shunned him. As a result of discussion with Kath, Michael developed an alternative perspective: 'If I need to use my inhaler in public people are unlikely to make a fuss, or ridicule or shun me'.

Behavioural experiments

Behavioural experiments

Behavioural experiments allow clients to test their beliefs in practical ways. They can take various forms, are precisely planned according to the belief that is being tested, and require creativity and ingenuity. For a guide to the development of behavioural experiments across a range of psychological problems, see Bennett-Levy *et al.* (2004). It is essential to adapt behavioural experiments with safety in mind, especially where an individual has a physical illness (see Wells, 1997, pp. 85 and 117, for further discussion).

For Michael it was important to evaluate his new ideas about how others might react if he used his inhaler in public. He agreed to test out his idea that 'If I need to use my inhaler in public people are unlikely to make a fuss, or ridicule or shun me'. He and Kath designed experiments to ascertain how people react to inhaler use. Firstly Michael would observe Kath using an inactive inhaler in a busy shopping centre. The prediction to be tested was that 'nobody will take any notice'. The experiment confirmed this and Michael then tested this out for himself with the same results. The next step was to use his inhaler in a variety of previously avoided, increasingly challenging situations. These behavioural experiments showed Michael that his fears were unfounded and that people reacted matter-of-factly to his inhaler use. Kath and Michael also talked about how Michael would respond if someone did ask him if he was OK or otherwise commented on his inhaler use. Possible scenarios were role-played in sessions. This work led to a reduction in the anxiety Michael felt when he became wheezy and to more prompt and effective self-medication. Finally Michael decided to talk to Karen about his asthma. He was concerned that she might react negatively but, following the work with Kath, decided this was unlikely. In the event she responded positively, telling him 'You are not your asthma'. This comment helped Michael realise that he had been placing undue emphasis on his asthma.

How might CBT be applied to help people with long-term conditions?

Using CBT in long-term conditions

CBT is increasingly being applied to problems of physical ill-health, particularly long-term conditions. There are several ways in which CBT can contribute to the care of people with such disorders:

- People with chronic ill-health (for example chronic pain or coronary heart disease) have increased vulnerability to developing common mental health problems such as depression and anxiety. These conditions may compromise the person's management of their physical problems. CBT is proven to be effective with such conditions. This application of CBT will be explored further in Chapter 8.
- Stress may directly or indirectly exacerbate long-term

conditions. CBT can assist patients to manage stress more effectively. Stress management techniques are discussed in Chapter 7.

- Individuals with long-term conditions face an unwelcome diagnosis with implications for the future. Adjusting to having a long-term condition may involve facing uncertainty and loss, for example of capacity and fitness, of the future that was envisaged before diagnosis and of a self-image as whole and healthy. Giving people opportunities to express and explore such feelings is important. CBT can provide a formulatory framework to help people understand the emotional impact of their condition. For further information see Bennett (1993) and Moorey (1996).

- Individuals have variable capacity to manage chronic ill health. People with very similar levels of physical impairment may have very different levels of disability (see Chapter 2). Beliefs about causation, nature, course, treatment and implications of an illness can influence how people respond to medical advice and manage illness. A CBT approach can promote improved understanding of health-related beliefs and more effective self-management. A cognitive–behavioural model of 'dysfunctional illness behaviour' in which self-schemas (encompassing a range of beliefs about self, the world and relationships) interact with beliefs about illness is presented by Williams (1997). These issues are addressed further in Chapters 3 and 4.

- For some conditions it may be desirable to make changes to exercise, diet, smoking, stress levels and so forth but change can be challenging for various reasons. Prochaska and DiClemente (1983) proposed that behaviour change follows a series of stages, which will be described further in Chapter 5. According to Rollnick *et al.* (1999) an individual's readiness to change depends on the perceived importance of making the change (taking into account possible benefits and costs) and their confidence in their ability to change. Where individuals are also struggling with some adversity or disadvantage (poverty, poor housing, single-parenthood, racism and so forth), the capacity to change may be compromised by competing concerns, lack of time or resources and reduced self-confidence. For further discussion of the clinical skills involved in behaviour change counselling, see Chapter 5.

Developing an effective helping relationship

Developing relationships

As noted earlier developing a therapeutic alliance based on respect, empathy and trust is essential to professional helping relationships. This is perhaps of particular importance when working with people with long-term conditions, for example, where the focus of consultation is change in health-relevant behaviour. There are numerous ways in which health professionals can inadvertently increase resistance to change, by giving advice in ways that restrict the client's sense of freedom and autonomy (often provoking a 'yes... but' response), failing to take account of the person's readiness to change or rushing ahead too rapidly and failing to understand the person's beliefs and knowledge about their condition.

The specific skills that characterise CBT (for example, guided discovery, including Socratic questioning, a collaborative stance and agenda setting) are relevant to behaviour change counselling. Rollnick *et al.* (1999, p. 78) in describing principles of good practice, emphasise the importance of taking an explicitly client-centred approach, focusing on the discovery of meaning:

> Ensure that the pace of the discussion is slowed down, and develop a genuine curiosity to know how this person really feels. You should listen to the answers to your questions, using techniques like reflection and other simple open questions to help patients express themselves as fully as possible. Your attention should not be on your own thought processes (e.g. What should I ask next?), but as much as possible on the meaning of what the person is saying. Trust the process and the patient.

CBT is explicitly collaborative. The therapist brings expertise and experience while the client is an expert in their own life. Implicit in CBT is the notion that the client can, with the therapist's assistance, find their own solutions. This is echoed by Rollnick *et al.* (1999, p. 75) who remind the reader: 'There is no sense in which you can be expected to have all the answers. Indeed you must believe that these lie mostly within the patient'. For further discussion of these and related issues, see Chapter 5.

The role of beliefs about illness (or 'illness representations')

Beliefs about illness

Beliefs about the identity, time-line, consequences, causes and potential cure or control of illness (Leventhal *et al.,* 1992) influence the management of long-term conditions. People with type 2 diabetes may have various beliefs about their condition. For example someone who believes that type 2 diabetes is less serious than type 1 may be less motivated to make appropriate lifestyle changes than someone who appreciates the condition's potential gravity. Further, someone with type 2 diabetes who believes they are well because they are asymptomatic may be similarly relaxed about lifestyle change. In contrast, a person who believes that type 2 is a serious but manageable condition may more readily perceive the importance of taking steps and be prepared to do so. Unhelpful beliefs for someone with coronary heart disease (CHD) might include the thought that exercise or anything else that increases their heart rate should be avoided because rapid heart beat signals imminent heart attack. The common sense model of illness behaviour (also referred to as the self-regulatory model of illness behaviour) (Leventhal *et al.,* 1992) describes how an individual's beliefs or illness representations about various aspects of illness can influence how the illness is managed. For further discussion of these issues see Chapters 3 and 4.

Self-monitoring

Self-monitoring, typically involving the use of a diary, is a core CBT technique, undertaken in the spirit of genuine curiosity – a desire to discover more about the problem. The form of the diary varies according to its focus. For example Michael learned more about his asthma management by keeping a diary. A person wishing to discover more about their eating habits might keep a diary something like that shown in Figure 1.3.

Figure 1.3

Eating habits diary

Date/time	Situation (when, where, with whom, etc.)	What did you eat/drink?

While it is important that the diary should not be overcomplicated, additional columns can be included to elicit further information. For example a person who describes eating when emotionally upset might record their thoughts and feelings prior to eating. Learning more about this pattern may be a first step towards identifying alternative strategies to cope with feelings such as boredom, anger, anxiety, sadness and so forth.

Numerous examples of diary formats can be found in cognitive therapy textbooks and CBT self-help publications. It is also useful to develop tailormade diaries collaboratively with clients. It is important to remember that self-monitoring can be a challenge, not least because it involves effort and can mean facing information about oneself that is surprising or unwelcome. The more the client is engaged in the process (for example helping design the diary), the more likely they are to keep records. It is also helpful to explore any potential barriers to keeping the diary and to use a problem-solving method (see Chapter 6) to develop solutions. For further information about diary use, see Chapters 6 and 9.

Exploring and identifying specific goals

Exploring goals

It is important to ask people what they themselves would like to achieve through their work with you. People may initially articulate goals that are general, e.g. 'I just want to feel better', or perhaps have no specific goal, e.g. 'I'm here because my doctor sent me'. In these instances it is helpful to clarify more specific, measurable goals, perhaps to lose weight, take more exercise or quit smoking. Goals may also centre on achieving change specific to a particular condition, for example to reduce blood pressure. Rollnick *et al.* (1999, p. 94) suggest that goal setting moves from the general to the specific. The steps involved are to identify a goal (e.g. to reduce blood pressure), to develop a strategy (e.g. to take more exercise) and identify specific targets involving behaviour change (e.g. walk to work, go swimming twice each week or attend a yoga class).

Negotiating goals may require the provision of information and feedback about results, for example a person with type 2 diabetes might be overweight and need to reduce this (e.g. moving from a

BMI (body mass index) of 32 to a BMI within the normal range), or they may need to understand the importance of foot care. Appropriate goals for someone with coronary heart disease might be smoking cessation or increasing the amount of exercise taken. Goal setting is discussed further in Chapter 6.

Points for reflection

- Spend some time thinking about the basic principles of CBT and how they relate to your personal experience. You might, for example, reflect on a recent time when you felt a shift in mood – anxiety, irritation, sadness, happiness, hope, etc. What was the situation? What thoughts went through your mind? How did these relate to your mood and behaviour? Did you notice any physical changes?

- Think about the difference between core beliefs, rules or assumptions and automatic thoughts. How would you describe these to a colleague?

- Consider the ways in which CBT principles assist the formation of a collaborative therapeutic alliance. How might you develop your own practice to incorporate these principles?

Chapter 2
Impairment and disability

Learning outcomes

By the end of this chapter you will be able to:
- briefly define impairment and disability
- understand how the relationship between impairment and disability works in people with a long-term condition
- explain the difference between the biomedical model and the biopsychosocial model.

Introduction

The care of people with long-term conditions has been a growing problem throughout the western world. Within the UK there are over 2 million people with diabetes (Diabetes UK, 2006), almost 9 million with arthritis (Mccormick *et al.*, 1995), up to 3 million with chronic obstructive pulmonary disease (Stang *et al.*, 2000), and 2.6 million living with heart disease (Petersen *et al.*, 2005). It has been estimated that in the county of Dorset and Somerset, which has a population of 1.2 million, it would take 23 years for three full-time general practioners to see each patient with a long-term condition once (Tomkins and Collins, 2006)! With these prevalence statistics it is not surprising that the UK Department of Health has been actively encouraging improved self-management for people with long-term conditions.

Self-management has been defined by Barlow *et al.*, 2002, p. 178 as:

> ...the individual's ability to manage the symptoms, treatment, physical and psychosocial consequences and life

style changes inherent in living with a chronic condition. Efficacious self-management encompasses ability to monitor one's condition and to effect the cognitive, behavioural and emotional responses necessary to maintain a satisfactory quality of life.

In a systematic review, Barlow *et al.* (2002) reported that people who learn to successfully self-manage their conditions report improvements in knowledge, behaviour, self-efficacy and health status. The same paper also stated that '...there is a need to train health professionals to ensure that patients' self-management abilities are maintained and fostered in clinical settings'. (Barlow *et al.*, 2002, p. 178)

This book aims to provide the knowledge and skills needed by health professionals in order for them to help people successfully manage long-term conditions.

In the 1980s, the World Health Organization stated that when assessing a patient with a long-term condition you should do so on three different levels, considering:

- impairment
- disability, and
- handicap (Wood, 1980).

We will not be considering handicap any further, as it is affected more by societal impositions on people with a disability, rather than what they can do to help to manage their conditions. However, it is important to have an understanding of what we mean by impairment or disability and how they differ from each other. When reading each of the definitions try to think of someone you have cared for or are caring for who falls within this definition.

Impairment

Impairment

Impairment is '*any loss or abnormality of psychological, physiological or anatomical structure or function*' (Wood, 1980, pp. 27–9), that is to say, the extent to which the person's body is different from that of a person in perfect health – what doctors call 'the lesion'. Impairment is measured at the level of the organ. Examples are:

- joint destruction in rheumatoid arthritis

- blockage of the arteries from atherosclerosis
- loss of brain tissue following a stroke.

Disability

Disability

Disability is *'any restriction or lack (resulting from an impairment) of ability to perform an activity in the manner or within the range considered normal for a human being'* (Wood, 1980, pp. 27–9). For example:

- restricted ability on an exercise tolerance test
- difficulties with activities in daily life
- symptoms (e.g. pain, shortness of breath)
- anxiety or depression.

In short, anything that reduces a person's abilities or quality of life compared to their healthy peers. Disability is disturbances in function at the level of the person.

So what does this difference mean for people?

Disability vs impairment

In terms of helping individual people, substantial research has shown that there is a lot that we can do to reduce disability. Indeed, if the person makes sufficient change to their lifestyle it is possible to make an impact on the impairment and reduce the disease progression, for example, to regress coronary heart disease.

A classic misconception about disability and impairment is that *impairment causes disability – therefore the worse the impairment the worse the disability*. It is vital not to make judgements or jump to conclusions about what a person can achieve based on the extent of the impairment. In reality, for most long-term conditions (except those at the extremes of impairment) this relationship does not exist; impairment and disability are not closely related. The following example is from someone with cardiac disease but the principles can be applied to anyone with a long-term condition.

Someone with cardiac disease could be judged on the following degrees of impairment:

- 75 per cent stenosis of a coronary artery – this is a major blockage of the artery

- a 40 per cent ejection fraction – the ejection fraction is a measurement of the heart's efficiency and should be around 75–85 per cent

- a 15 per cent ejection fraction.

Based on these indicators (describing impairments) consider whether it would be possible to answer for each person the following questions (describing the disability experienced):

- How far could they walk?

- How much help would they need with activities of daily living?

- How anxious or depressed would they be?

- How much pain would they report?

- How often would they be admitted to hospital?

In reality it is impossible to answer these questions with the information given, which illustrates the point that impairment does not relate to disability.

A direct relationship between any two factors such as height and weight, would be shown in a graph as a relatively straight line. We can create height and weight charts that roughly fit most people, but we can never measure impairment and then deduce how disabled a person will be. If there was a direct relationship between impairment and disability the results would look like the graph in Figure 2.1. Reading across the graph, low impairment is associated with low disability, and high impairment with high disability.

Figure 2.1 **Expected relationship between impairment and disability**

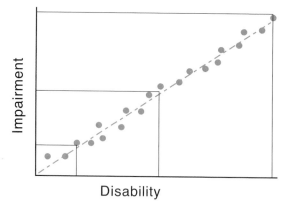

Compare this with the graph in Figure 2.2, which is taken from a real study. It shows the actual relationship between the amount of work a person could perform on an exercise test and their ejection fraction.

Figure 2.2

Actual relationship between impairment and disability (in people with heart failure)

Courtesy of David Hare

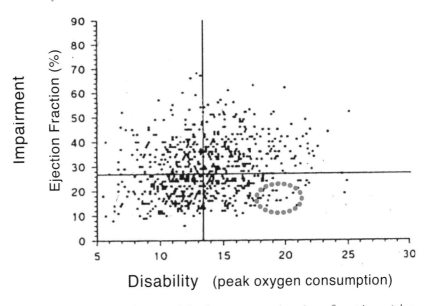

If there was a relationship between ejection fraction (the impairment) and the amount people in the study could do on a treadmill (peak VO_2 – the disability), then the dots would form a straight line as in Figure 2.1. It is clear that there is no relationship between the impairment and disability. The scatter plot is essentially random, or to put it another way, the ejection fraction tells you absolutely nothing about how much the patient can do. Some people with an ejection fraction between 10 per cent and 20 per cent and thus with a severely impaired heart (dotted circle on the graph above) were able to do a great deal more work than others with an ejection fraction between 40 per cent and 70 per cent (mild to moderate impairment).

Although we have used the ejection fraction and exercise capacity as the example here, it is true with other impairments:

- **Respiratory disease** – lung function tests such as forced expiratory volume show a poor correlation with breathlessness, which is often better measured by health status questionnaires (Jones *et al.*, 1992).

- **Angina** – the level of blockage of the arteries will not tell you how much angina the person experiences or how disabled they are by the angina (Smith *et al.,* 1984).

- **Functional bowel disorders** – the severity of pain is better predicted by psychological factors such as depression than by physiological assessment of the bowel (Drossman *et al.,* 2000).

- **Myocardial infarction (MI)** – the size of an infarct in the average MI patient will not tell you how anxious or depressed they will become, whether they will return to work, or how it will affect the rest of their life (Beck *et al.,* 2001, Lane *et al.,* 2000).

We all know some people whose medical findings suggest that they should be bed-bound and yet live a near-normal life and, in contrast, other people who have little wrong with their bodies yet live like invalids.

The message we need to keep in mind is: *Never guess what a person can or can't achieve on the basis of their impairment.*

There is only one way to find out what a person can achieve over time. *Help them to use goal setting and see how far they can get.* Goal setting and other tools are discussed in detail later in the book.

Why is impairment not related to disability?

Psychologists have studied this strange fact for a number of years and although they do not understand all of the reasons, they do understand some. The good news is that some of the factors that lead to people becoming more disabled have been identified and can be changed. This knowledge is the basis of cognitive–behavioural disease management programmes.

The following pages illustrate two contrasting case stories that may also help to provide insights into why people may start with a similar degree of impairment but end up with different degrees of disability.

Case example 2

Omar

Omar had worked hard and was looking forward to enjoying his retirement with his wife, Yasmeen, helping to care for his grandchildren. Shortly before retiring, he was admitted to hospital with a heart attack. At first, this frightened him greatly. After he was discharged, he spent quite a lot of time looking for information to find out what changes he needed to make to get control over his illness.

- His job had involved sitting at a desk so he was largely inactive.
- Both he and Yasmeen loved to eat (she was a fantastic cook), which was probably why they were both overweight.
- He had smoked for years.
- He had been diagnosed with diabetes a couple of years ago.

He could see that all of these problems had led to the heart attack and most importantly that each could be remedied or controlled; this helped to settle his anxiety a little. Like many people, initially he blamed stress for his heart attack, mainly because of his work but also because he was 'always a great worrier'. His whole family also believed this and tried to protect him from any excitement or work.

'Omar, don't do that, you'll overtire yourself.'

'Granddad, you just sit and rest, we'll get you a drink of coffee.'

His family wouldn't even let him play with little Ahmed, his boisterous grandson, saying that the play might get out of hand and be too much for him.

This became much less of a problem when he was introduced to a health worker who discussed these ideas with him and Yasmeen. The health worker explained that they were common but unhelpful misconceptions and that the truth was the reverse, that it was important for him to do more, not less, if he wanted to be protected from further problems. The health worker showed him how to set goals and how to work towards these goals in a systematic and safe manner.

Over the next year, with his wife's help, he tackled his diet and he and Yasmeen began to take a daily walk. This was slowly extended until after a few months they walked for an hour or so every day. They both lost weight and felt fitter than they had in years. He also gained good control of his blood sugar.

He had had a few episodes of angina when he first got out of hospital, which had made him very anxious. His health worker found he had a number of misconceptions about angina, believing that it was a kind of 'mini heart attack' for example. This had made him frightened to do anything that might bring it on. His health worker discussed this and reassured him that angina, unlike a heart attack, does not damage the heart. As a result of all of the changes he'd made his angina never reappeared.

He and Yasmeen now had the active retirement of which they had dreamed. To use their own words, 'they were at the best part of their life'. People who met them had no inkling that he had had a heart attack, indeed they often commented on his energy level and how well he looked for his age.

Case example 3

Graham

Graham lived with his wife Sarah in the same town as Omar and Yasmeen. Like Omar, Graham had just retired from a desk job. He was admitted to the same ward on the same day as Omar, with a similar myocardial infarction and they were discharged on the same day, which is how they met and became friends.

Graham had known other people who had had heart attacks, so he had been able to tell Omar how careful they both needed to be. He had many misconceptions, for example:

● another heart attack must be just around the corner

● stress and excitement are very dangerous for a person with a weak heart

● angina would damage his heart.

To protect his heart Graham didn't do anything that he thought might bring on angina. If an activity did provoke any chest pain or even breathlessness, he stopped doing it. The hobbies he had planned to take up when he retired, fishing and sailing, were definitely off the agenda. He had been involved in town life before his heart attack but dropped this afterwards and somehow never felt quite well enough to get back to it.

He became more and more dependent on Sarah and this didn't help the way he felt about himself. He felt like he had gone from being the breadwinner and supporter of his family to being dependent and no longer respected. He became angry, snapped at people, had poor sleep and multiple aches and pains that the doctor seemed unable to diagnose or cure. In his black moments, he had begun to think that the doctor had given up on him because his case was medically hopeless, because all he had been offered was to see a counsellor – nothing to do with his heart!

Sarah was stressed too. The heart attack had made her feel helpless and guilty that she had let him become overweight; alarmingly this was getting worse. She felt all she could do was protect Graham and try to reassure him. If she mentioned eating less he flared up, saying it was the only pleasure he had left. It was very tiring trying to do everything that Graham had once done, as well as look after the house. The grandchildren weren't allowed to make any noise when they came over, so they visited less and less. Sarah was becoming increasingly depressed, and was often quite angry with Graham, but she didn't dare to argue with him in case it caused another heart attack.

After six months Graham was very overweight, his blood pressure was out of control and he was taking a number of medicines, some of which left him feeling tired and ill; he had developed type 2 diabetes. He got lots of advice from doctors and nurses and often resolved to 'lose weight and try to take more exercise' as he had been advised. Twice he went for a long walk only to have to call a taxi, once from someone's house and then from a phone box, because he was exhausted. Graham and Sarah often said how much luckier Omar had been than Graham, whose life had become dominated by the illness. Graham's family all agreed that Omar's heart attack must have been a very small one or maybe not a heart attack at all!

Graham and Omar were lying side by side in the coronary care unit with drips in their arms – they were both equally disabled. As the days and weeks went by their level of disability began to diverge, until a year later they could not present a more complete contrast even though their underlying impairment was the same.

Omar had successfully managed his illness and was a picture of health and well-being. Graham had become an invalid, anxious and depressed with strained family relation-ships, a rotten quality of life and a rapidly increasing risk of further medical problems.

Our job is to ensure, as far as possible, that the potential Grahams end up like Omar. The rest of this book will explain how.

Why do Omar and Graham show different levels of disability?

In order to understand the differences between Omar and Graham, we need to look at the factors that may contribute to the development of different levels of disability in people with similar long-term conditions.

Many years of research, by many people, show that in a long-term condition the amount of impairment cannot, on its own, explain:

- the extent (or lack of) disability
- the extent of the symptoms reported
- the success or failure of medical treatment or surgery
- the number of acute medical events and readmissions
- medical costs (Lewin, 1997).

In order to be able to explain the above factors, you also need to know and understand:

- the person's beliefs about their illness
- the person's own attempts to cope
- psychological features, such as motivation and self-efficacy
- the person's level of anxiety and depression
- the degree of social support and their social class (Lewin, 1997).

A number of these: beliefs, coping attempts, motivation, self-efficacy and anxiety and depression, are all things that can be changed using cognitive–behavioural methods.

Figure 2.3 **Levels of disability in people with the same degree of impairment**

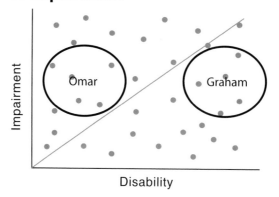

Figure 2.3 illustrates how your role as a clinician is to help people to behave more like Omar, i.e. less disabled than their impairment suggests they should be, and less like Graham, i.e. more disabled than their impairment suggests they need to be.

Biomedical and biopsychosocial models of illness

Models of illness

So far in this chapter we have contrasted the biomedical view of disability whereby *impairment causes disability* with a biopsychosocial view of disability, that impairment, the biological difference between people, is only one factor and that *disability is the result of an interaction between biological, psychological and social factors.* Figure 2.4 shows the biomedical model.

Figure 2.4

The biomedical model of disease

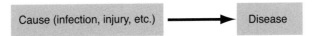

The biopsychosocial model is a way of looking at the mind and body of a person as a whole. The model was developed by psychiatrist George Engel in a 1977 article in *Science* (Engel, 1977). Engel proposed that:

> ... a model should take into account the patient, the social context in which he lives, and the complementary system devised by society to deal with the disruptive effects of illness, that is, the physician role and the health care system. This requires a biopsychosocial model.

Engel based the biopsychosocial model on von Bertanlaffy's application of general systems theory to molecular biology, which proposes that all levels of organisation (from molecular level to societal levels) are linked to illness. Illness and disease do not necessarily run together. A person may be reasonably well (with no sickness), but if they feel unwell that's an illness. Similarly, people with something physically wrong with them are diseased, but they may feel completely all right – they are not ill. This relates back to the disability versus impairment debate described previously.

The biopsychosocial model gives greater importance to the illness, rather than the disease, and therefore much more information needs to be gathered during a consultation. As well as the biological signs and symptoms, it is important to find out about the person's psychological state, their feelings and beliefs and their hierarchical relationship; therefore change in one component of the model will result in change in the other components (von Bertanlaffy, 1975).

The model draws a distinction between the actual pathological processes that cause disease and the person's perception of their health and the effects on it, called the illness/disease, and social factors such as their relationship with their families and the larger community.

Compare the biomedical model and the biopsychosocial model in Figures 2.4 and 2.5.

Figure 2.5   **The biopsychosocial model of illness experience**

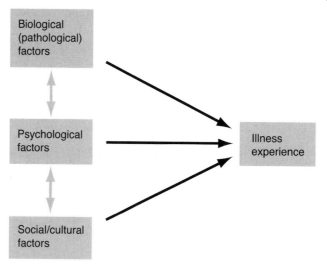

Unfortunately, many of the interactions we as health workers have with people are conducted from a biomedical perspective. This means that we act as if all of the outcomes can be explained by the physical aspects of the disease – anatomy, physiology, biochemistry and pathology. Although this perspective has been very useful for finding the underlying physiological causes of disease and impairment, we now know that this narrow perspective can be very unhelpful when applied to people with a long-term condition.

We would argue that in its 'true' meaning, health is more than just *not having* a disease. It is a positive state of well-being.

Compare Omar and Graham; both have the same amount of disease in their coronary arteries yet, in their own estimation and that of others, one is 'healthy', the other an invalid. Ignoring this wider definition of health and concentrating on the biomedical aspects alone can lead to poor outcomes for people, frustration with health workers and unexplained results such as 'The operation was a success; unfortunately the patient is no better'.

The following cases illustrate examples of a biomedically and a biopsychosocially orientated consultation.

Case example 4

John – a biomedically orientated consultation

John had received treatment for a broken leg and was having some difficulty in getting back to work, so he went to see his doctor. The conversation went like this:

Doctor: Hello John, sit down just there. How's the leg? You should be just about ready to go back to work, shouldn't you?

John: Well doctor, my leg still aches a lot. The physio tells me that I should do more but I can't. I don't know when I'm going to be fit for work. It's getting me down, I can tell you.

Doctor: Well, I'll sign you off for another week. Have you got enough painkillers? Listen to your body, and work with that, but do try to do the exercises that the physio set. They won't work unless you put some effort into them.

John: Thanks doctor, I'll try. I could do with some more painkillers. When do you want to see me again?

Doctor: Next week. See you then.

John was been signed off work for another week and was given a prescription for painkillers. Is this how it should be? Did the doctor miss something? Below are a couple of points for reflection based on what we have talked about so far.

Points for reflection

- Are there any points that John made which you would like more information on?
- What do you think of the advice about exercise?

We can use the biopsychosocial model to analyse what happened in the consultation in Case example 4.

Case example 4 revisited

Doctor: Hello John, sit down just there. How's the leg? [*The doctor focuses immediately on the impairment, the break in the bone, not the human being.*] You should be just about ready to go back to work, shouldn't you? [*He makes assumptions about John's state of health based on the expected time for a broken bone to mend.*]

John: Well doctor, my leg still aches a lot. The physio tells me that I should do more but I can't. I don't know when I'm going to be fit for work. It's getting me down, I can tell you.

Doctor: Well I'll sign you off for another week. Have you got enough painkillers? [*The doctor perceives that the aching leg is nothing to worry about, so ignores it. John doesn't seem to be doing what the physiotherapist is advising him to do, so he thinks 'I should encourage him to be compliant'*] Listen to your body, and work with that, but try to do the exercises that the physio set. [*He thinks 'I'll have to sign him off for another week; hopefully he'll comply with treatment next week – not much else I can do'*]

John: Thanks doctor. I could do with some more painkillers. When do you want to see me again?

Doctor: Next week; see you then.

Being without work for a long time may impact on John's finances and his relationship with his relatives, reduce his social life and cause further anxiety and depression. Continuing with painkillers can lead to unwanted side effects or dependency. This can all lead to a downward spiral of increasing disability.

Case example 5 shows another perspective on the consultation if the biopsychosocial approach had been adopted. The doctor uses a number of techniques that are explained in the chapters that follow.

Case example 5

John – doing it the biopsychosocial way

Doctor: Hello John, please take a seat. What have you come to see me about?

John: It's about my leg doctor; my leg still aches a lot. The physio tells me that I should be able to do more but I can't. I don't know when I should be ready for work. It's getting me down, I can tell you.

Doctor: So you are worried about your leg, because it is still very sore. Let's talk about that for a minute – we'll come back to your exercises and returning to work afterwards. Tell me about the aches. When do they come on and what are they like?

John: Well, when I do anything I get an ache. Some days I feel absolutely fine, no problems at all. There are other times when the ache is really bad; all I can do is lie on the sofa with my feet up. My wife and kids have to wait on me because I can't do anything and they are getting a bit hacked off with it. I think that they are starting to think that I am faking it, but I'm not. I need to get back to work as the debts are mounting and I'm really worried.

Doctor: Being off work has caused money problems that are worrying you, and the ache in your leg comes and goes so that your family don't seem to believe you have a problem, is that it?

John: In a nutshell, yes.

Doctor: Tell me about what happens on a day when you feel fine, and have no ache in your leg. What can you do?

John: I can do anything. It's great. I catch up on things I haven't done, and I do all of the exercises that the physio showed me, even the hard ones. I can go out with the family for a walk or a bike ride – it's great! But as I said, when the leg is aching I can't do anything. I have to rest.

Doctor: So you do lots on good days and have to rest on bad days? It sounds like you have been trying hard to overcome your problem and get better. Can you think of any reason why you have bad days? Is there any pattern to it?

John: I hadn't thought of it like that, but I suppose there might be. If I think about it, I think my leg really plays up the day after I've given it a really good workout. Is that what's happened – I've been overdoing things?

Doctor: One way that we can find out is for you to keep a diary of your activities for a week, and to record how your leg feels each day. That way you may be able to see a pattern, and work out how much you can do safely without making your leg hurt.

John: I'll do that; it would be good to be able to do something.

Doctor: Once you know what you can do without pain, you can gradually increase the amount you do to get your leg a bit fitter. The main thing is to make the increases small so you don't overdo it again and your fitness and confidence return.

John: That would be great, to get better and see a light at the end of the tunnel.

Doctor: About your exercises – why do you think that you are having a problem with them?

John: Now I've talked to you I think it may be I've been doing them wrong. The physio told me to start with the easier exercises and work up to the harder ones but I thought the easy ones were too easy, so, when my leg felt okay, I would do the hard ones as often as I could. I can give them another go, and do them properly, just starting with the easy ones and working up – just like you said.

This case illustrates how using the biopsychosocial model makes a difference. It is clear that at the end of this consultation there is a different outcome and experience for John than in the biomedical case study.

The role of the patient's own perceptions

The patient's perceptions

In the biomedical model the focus is only on the disease; in the biopsychosocial view the person's perceptions of their health are also important in the 'illness experience'. How a person feels or thinks about their health may seem irrelevant but compare Graham and Omar; one life was dominated by ill health, the other by good health.

Many people have changes in their body that are 'disease' processes, for example, silent coronary artery disease is almost 'normal' in some western settings in men of 65. Yet the great majority live a normal 'healthy life' and see themselves as perfectly healthy, saying 'I've never had a day's illness in my life!', or 'I'm as strong as an ox!'. What would happen if due to some (imaginary) screening policy half of the 65-year-olds were suddenly told they have heart disease or diabetes? It is our contention that a proportion of these people would become, like Graham, disabled.

It may seem that all this is unnecessarily philosophical but because health is dependent not only on the biological evidence but also on a person's own perceptions, we too must take their perceptions into account and regard good health as more complicated than simply being *disease free*. It is probable that a proportion of people who appear to be disabled by 'ill health' will have no discernable lesion.

Points for reflection

- Consider impairment and disability – having read this chapter, think about how you would describe each of these to a colleague.

- Consider how you might explain whether or not there is a relationship between impairment and disability.

- Think about whether or not you can absolutely judge the amount of disability a person will have based on a measure of impairment.

- Reflect on the difference in the doctor's language and type of questions used in the case studies of the different models.

- Think about a recent consultation you have undertaken – replay it in your mind. What model did you use?

Chapter 3
Unhelpful patient beliefs

Learning outcomes

By the end of this chapter you will be able to:

- describe how beliefs about an illness can affect how people cope with it
- understand how specific misconceptions about living with a long-term condition affect behaviour, anxiety and depression.

Introduction

People can become anxious as a result of having a long-term condition. They may also change the way they live their lives because of misunderstandings about their condition. The following five factors contribute to how disabled a person with a long-term condition will be:

- anxiety and depression
- coping ability
- psychological factors
- family context and social support
- beliefs.

This chapter explores beliefs about health and illness. You may remember from Chapter 2, that Omar coped very well after his heart attack but Graham did not. One of the reasons that they coped so differently is that they held very different beliefs about what had happened to them and what they should do about it. Table 3.1 lists of some of the most common beliefs about heart disease. Write down whether you think they are right or wrong. We'll look at the answers later.

Chronic disease management for long-term conditions

Table 3.1   **Patient beliefs about heart disease**

Beliefs	Right or wrong?
One of the main causes of heart disease is stress	
Rest is the best medicine for heart conditions	
Heart disease is often caused by people's lifestyle	
Angina is a kind of small heart attack	
Once you have had one heart attack you are bound to have another	
People with angina should live life to the full	

So why is this important? It is vital as health workers that:

- we recognise that people all arrive with different beliefs about health and illness

- we use language and explanations that help people see their condition in a way that is meaningful to them and that does not reinforce misconceptions about health and illness.

Common-sense model of illness

A theoretical model that attempts to explain how beliefs interact with behaviour is Leventhal's common sense model of illness behaviour (Leventhal *et al.*, 1980, Leventhal *et al.*, 1997). The model (Figure 3.1) has three stages:

Stage 1

People interpret their symptoms to try to work out what is wrong. This is influenced by what they already know as well as information from sources such as nurses, doctors, friends, family, acquaintances and the media.

Their explanation will include ideas about what the illness is, what caused it, how long it is likely to last, whether it can be cured or controlled, and the consequences of having it. These thoughts will produce an emotional response (Leventhal and Cameron, 1987, Petrie *et al.*, 1996,). For example, if someone believes that they have a serious illness with no cure they are likely to be frightened (Hagger and Orbell, 2003).

Leventhal *et al.* (1992) propose two parallel pathways in the

Figure 3.1

Common-sense model of illness behaviour
(After Leventhal *et al.*, 1980 and 1992, reproduced with permission.)

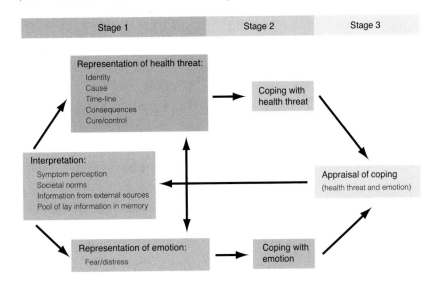

formation of an illness representation. The first is based on memories of illness (schematic) taken from direct illness experience. The second is based on memories about illness (conceptual or propositional knowledge). Memory of illness is arguably more persuasive than the abstract conceptual or theoretical knowledge one holds about illness. Leventhal *et al.*, (1992) illustrate this with the example of a nurse with hypertension who, while having the theoretical knowledge that it is impossible to tell whether blood pressure is raised through changes in bodily state (symptoms), nonetheless checks her blood pressure when headaches occur. Finding it raised, she takes medication accordingly (memory of illness), so reinforcing her idea that she can detect hypertension. Leventhal *et al.*, (1992) suggest that it can be difficult for people to integrate these two types of knowledge and that illness representations derived from direct experience can feel more convincing. The paper discusses the implications of the common sense model for helping people manage illness more effectively. Giving patients the space to explore illness representations relevant to their condition and its management is an important step in facilitating effective self-management.

Stage 2

Once the person has a representation of the illness in their minds, they will think about what they can do about it (coping) (Leventhal *et al., 1997*; Petrie *et al., 1996*). For example, if they believe that they can control the illness they are more likely to make an effort to change. If they believe that there is nothing they can do, they may become passive and simply try to avoid anything that could make the problem worse (Hagger and Orbell, 2003).

Stage 3

People constantly re-evaluate to see if they are succeeding and if their chosen action is helping. This feeds back into their beliefs which can change as a result.

This model is only one suggestion as to what determines how people will behave when they have an illness and there are several other slightly different competing models. The debate as to which is most accurate will no doubt continue for many decades. However this model illustrates that it is possible for us to think about how people's behaviour comes about.

All mainstream models of health behaviour share the assumption that the actions we take are the result of beliefs, knowledge and thought. It is obvious that if some thoughts and beliefs are correct and help us behave in ways that improve our health, others may work in the opposite way and lead to behaviours that cause poorer health. The beliefs that can hinder recovery have been studied and in cardiac illnesses are called cardiac misconceptions. A central part of the health worker's role can be to help people identify and then change these misconceptions.

The evidence around misconceptions

Evidence on mis- conceptions

It should be noted that the majority of evidence for the effect of specific misconceptions is exclusive to heart disease; little research has been undertaken in other disease areas. While misconceptions have been reported in other chronic illnesses (for example, the Diabetes UK website has a section about myths), the effects of these specific misconceptions have not been researched in the way that they have for heart disease. So people do have misconceptions about other long-term conditions and it is still an important concept to consider and be aware of when supporting anyone with a long-term condition.

In 1961, the National Heart Foundation of Australia established a Work Assessment Centre to help in the prevention and treatment of unnecessary invalidism of patients with heart disease. The centre assessed and interviewed 400 patients who had not returned to work after a heart attack. Of the 400 patients, 50 per cent were found to have emotional distress and invalidism that was not warranted by the extent of their illness, or by psychological, social and economic factors that would normally be expected and that were unavoidable (Wynn, 1967).

It was found that people who suffered undue anxiety adopted an over-cautious lifestyle, often taking early retirement because they believed that work was harmful. It was also found that anxiety was often caused or increased by remarks made by the medical and nursing staff. Table 3.2 shows some examples of the remarks from health workers, and the way that the patients interpreted them, taken from the study by Wynn (1967).

Table 3.2

Common misinterpretations of health workers' comments

Health workers' remarks	Patients' interpretations
'Lie still and you'll be alright'	'Move and I will die'
'You will be alright if you are careful'	'If I am not careful I'll die'
'You were lucky this time'	'I won't be so lucky next time'
'You haven't had a heart attack this time'	'A heart attack was imminent'

There were further misconceptions about the anatomy and physiology of the heart and how it had been affected by the heart attack: 'Half my heart is dead and the other half is dying', 'The main artery to my heart is blocking up' (Wynn, 1967, p. 849).

Furthermore many people interpreted their own symptoms incorrectly, believing that each attack of angina was a fresh but smaller heart attack. Partners were often more confused than the patients because of lack of education and support from the health workers. Many wives had been told in the first days of the myocardial infarction that their husband might die, and had not since been told that the risk was now reduced. Consequently, the wives were overprotective and unduly fearful. People often believed that returning to work would cause further heart problems (Wynn, 1967).

Further studies of the effects of cardiac misconceptions have shown that people with more misconceptions are more anxious, depressed and physically limited, less likely to return to work and more likely to have unnecessary admissions to hospital (Maeland and Havik, 1989; Furze *et al.*, 2001, 2003). It has also been demonstrated that reducing the number of misconceptions held by people with heart disease was a better predictor of improvement in physical functioning than reducing their angina symptoms (Furze *et al.*, 2005).

It is important when a pathological or medical explanation for a disease process is given that it is balanced by an explanation that includes information in a way that does not reinforce or introduce misconceptions. This is why it is so important to understand an individual's beliefs about health and illness.

Evidence for interventions to reduce cardiac misconceptions

One of the first attempts to help cardiac patients reassess their cardiac misconceptions was *The Heart Manual* (Lewin *et al.*, 1992). In a randomised controlled trial patients either worked through *The Heart Manual* with brief phone support from a health worker, or they received a bundle of literature about heart disease, diet, smoking, exercise and so on from authoritative sources plus an equal amount of phone contact from the facilitator, during which their questions were answered and they were encouraged in their efforts to recover.

At 12 months the people who had carried out *The Heart Manual* programme were less anxious and depressed, had a better quality of life and had been admitted to hospital only half as often as the information and counselling patients (Lewin *et al.*, 1992).

A hospital-based programme, the Angina Management Programme, was also developed on a cognitive–behavioural understanding, and attempts to change misconceptions reduced angina by 70 per cent, reducing disability, anxiety and depression. Half of those patients who had been awaiting bypass surgery were so much better that their cardiologist advised them there was no point in the surgery and they were removed from the list (Lewin *et al.*, 1995).

The Angina Management Programme has been turned into a

home-based programme called *The Angina Plan*. In a randomised controlled trial in primary care, when compared to a 'usual' nurse-led angina clinic, it reduced angina by 40 per cent while leaving patients much more active and reducing anxiety and depression (Lewin *et al.,* 2002).

Others have adopted similar cognitive approaches. In New Zealand a health psychologist, Keith Petrie, examined the effect of a brief hospital-based intervention delivered by a psychologist. It was based around Leventhal's illness behaviour model and was designed to change health beliefs. The intervention was compared to routine, nurse-directed standard care in a randomised study of 65 patients. At three-month follow-up, the intervention group had significantly more positive views about their myocardial infarction, had returned to work more quickly and had fewer bouts of angina (Petrie *et al.,* 2002).

Myths about heart disease

Myths about heart disease

At the beginning of the chapter we asked you to answer a few questions, some of which were misconceptions. Table 3.3 lists the answers.

Table 3.3

Beliefs about heart disease – the truths

Belief about heart disease	Right or wrong?
One of the main causes of heart disease is stress	Wrong
Rest is the best medicine for heart conditions	Wrong
Heart disease is often caused by people's lifestyle	Right
Angina is a kind of small heart attack	Wrong
Once you have had one heart attack you are bound to have another	Wrong
People with angina should live life to the full	Right

So far we have explained that wrong ideas or misconceptions may lead to unhelpful coping actions which can lead to worsening of health in its broadest sense. To go right back to the start, this might help to explain why disability is often not related to the extent of the disease. It may also explain why people with mistaken ideas have more symptoms and are admitted to hospital more often. Finally it may explain why some people are more anxious than others.

The examples used in this chapter are taken from questionnaires of misconceptions about living with heart disease. In Chapter 9 on assessment and outcome we include more detail on how to assess people's beliefs about their long-term condition using such questionnaires.

Listening and observing to spot misconceptions

Spotting misconceptions

Although using a beliefs questionnaire will trap some of the more common misconceptions, people may still not make the connection between how they are behaving and their underlying beliefs about disease.

Case example 6

Steve

This is an example from a home visit by Sally, a health worker, to Steve who has chronic respiratory disease and has just been discharged home following a hospital admission for pneumonia. It's a nice sunny day, so Steve invites Sally into the garden to drink tea.

Sally: This is a wonderful garden that you've got.

Steve: I think it does look great, full of flowers in bloom at different times of the year, because I'm a keen gardener. But now with my chest problems getting so much worse we've been thinking of getting some men in to cut it down and have it all put down to grass. That way I could keep on top of it with as I've got one of those ride-on mowers.

Sally: Is that what you really want to do?

Steve: No, I love gardening, but my wife isn't strong and she couldn't do all of the pruning and digging. And I can't do that either now.

Sally: What made you decide you couldn't do your gardening anymore?

Steve: Well I don't know if I could but I need to be careful, even the doctor in the hospital said that.

Sally: I think he meant not smoking and keeping your weight down. We also know that people who keep up with their exercise can also help their breathing. How much gardening did you do that was really hard?

Steve: I hadn't really thought about it, but most of the time it is more pottering about, you know, a bit of gentle hoeing, dead-heading the flowers, things like that. I suppose because most of the garden is mature there isn't as much heavy digging any more.

Sally: I think that you are really lucky because sitting out there you've got your own gym and you enjoy working in it!

Steve: So you are telling me it is quite safe and I can go back to doing everything I used to do? I was really frightened that I would become so breathless that I would end up back in hospital.

Sally: We know that it is a lot safer to be active than it is to sit around. What we can do is to set some activity goals with your garden that can help to increase your fitness, so that you don't get too breathless. In the meantime, would your son-in-law be willing to help with some of the more strenuous tasks until we get your fitness back to where it was?

Steve: I'm sure he'd be very glad to help. And I wouldn't mind him doing it if I knew it was only for a while, until I got stronger. Sally, you've made my day, I feel brighter already.

Steve had indicated to Sally in a previous discussion that you should 'live life to the full' but he clearly didn't think that included gardening. He, and possibly his family (notice the use of 'we' in 'we've been thinking of getting some men in to it cut down') still had misconceptions about the effect of work on his respiratory disease. Sally asked whether this was what he really wanted to do, which led to her discovery of his underlying misconception that 'over-doing it' in the garden could lead to further problems.

When a person reports giving up or avoiding anything, especially those things that they used to enjoy, it is important to check why. It can be the way in to a very useful discussion that reveals many misconceptions.

Changing misconceptions

Changing misconceptions

Sometimes it is enough to tell a person that their belief is wrong. Often, though, more is required to balance folklore, anxiety in the person, misunderstandings of things said in hospital and the influence of the person's friends and family. If you simply contradict the person's beliefs you may arouse resistance. Later in the book we explain about health behaviour change counselling (developed from motivational interviewing) and different ways to help patients become aware of their health beliefs and alter them where necessary.

Rollnick *et al*. (1999), (see Chapter 6) describe a three-stage process of information exchange. The first step is to elicit the person's readiness and interest in learning more about the condition (e.g. What is your understanding of...?) and to ascertain if they would like further information (e.g. Would you like to know more about...?). Following Leventhal *et al*. (1992) it is arguably also important to explore the person's experience of the illness.

The second stage is to provide information or feedback in a neutral manner, in language the patient can understand and at a suitable pace. Finally the impact of this new information is elicited (e.g. What do you make of this...?). Here points of difference between schematic and conceptual memories may be explored. In discussing the case of the nurse with conflicting beliefs about blood pressure, Leventhal *et al*. (1992, p. 149) suggest that '...we might alter the nurse's confidence in her symptoms as reliable indicators of blood pressure... if she finds that her pressure is elevated when she is asymptomatic'. Once a representation has been altered a behavioural change would need to follow, in this case to find an alternative cue for taking medication. This process follows CBT principles of guided discovery. An illustration is given opposite.

Case example 7

Margaret

Margaret, a retired sales executive in her 60s, suffered a heart attack. Her husband called an ambulance and she received prompt and effective treatment, making a good recovery. Since her heart attack she avoids all but the most minimal exertion and has become fearful of emotional stress. Over time her quality of life and her fitness have deteriorated. Her husband is concerned about her and has taken on more and more household and other tasks. Prior to the heart attack she and her husband were enjoying an active retirement. Margaret's cardiac rehabilitation nurse, Anne, has become concerned about Margaret's dejected mood and her self-reported fear about engaging in any physically or emotionally stressful activity. Anne thinks it would be helpful to find out more about Margaret's understanding of her CHD and her beliefs about exercise.

Anne: How have you been getting on since we last met?

Margaret: Not too good really. I haven't felt up to doing much but I feel guilty that Bob is having to do so much around the house. I get fed up and then I get snappy with him which is unfair. I also feel worried when I get upset because I think 'this is putting stress on your heart, you'll bring on another heart attack'. Last week I felt really stressed with it all and afraid and trapped. I started to feel shaky and clammy, my heart started to beat faster and I got really scared that I was going to have a heart attack. Bob actually called the ambulance but when I got to hospital they said my symptoms were anxiety and sent me home. I felt terrible, like a real time-waster.

Anne: That must have been very upsetting for you. What did you make of what the doctor said?

Margaret: I wasn't convinced but then Bob made me a cup of tea at home and I watched some TV and things sort of settled down so I suppose it couldn't have been a heart attack. And yet at the time I was sure it was. I was terrified.

Anne: That must feel confusing. On the one hand feeling upset leads to symptoms you associate with a heart attack. On the other hand the doctor assures you that it's anxiety.

Margaret: Well yes, it is confusing. I don't know what to do for the best. And because my job was so stressful I sort of think 'well maybe that caused the heart attack'. Now I try to avoid any sort of stress or anything that makes my heart beat fast.

Anne: How does that affect your feelings about the home exercise programme we discussed?

Margaret: Well I've not done it except at the start. The first couple of times my heart started to beat faster and I know you said that was OK as long as I stuck to the programme and took it step by step but it just reminded me of having the heart attack and I got scared and stopped. I thought 'what if I'd carried on?' and saw myself being rushed to hospital again. I know I should be doing what I can to get fit so I don't have another attack and what you said about gentle exercise made sense. The trouble is when I find my heart rate increasing I get really frightened and that sort of takes over.

Anne: That memory is very powerful for you and it makes sense that you would want to do everything possible to avoid another heart attack. It sounds as if although you understand the reasons for the programme you become very worried when you feel your heart rate increasing.

Margaret: That's exactly it.

Following Leventhal *et al.* (1992) Margaret's concerns are understandable. For someone who has experienced a heart attack their memory of illness may include a frightening increase in heart rate. Conceptual level knowledge (memory about illness) regarding the benefits of exercise that elevates heart rate, may be less persuasive in the face of a powerful and emotionally charged memory. The implication of such a belief might be to regard with fear or scepticism any exercise-based cardiac rehabilitation programme, leading to poorer outcome. Exploring such beliefs in a non-judgemental way and offering information as appropriate will be important in helping Margaret.

Anne asks Margaret if it would be helpful to have more information about the role of exercise in managing coronary heart disease and also about the physical effects of anxiety. In addition, as Margaret is worried about the effects of emotional stress on her heart, Anne tells her about a stress management group that her service runs. On this course Margaret will learn more about stress and ways to manage it more effectively. At the next session Margaret asks if Bob can join them. They talk about the differences between anxiety symptoms and heart attack symptoms and Bob is able to express his worries about Margaret and explore why he has taken over so many household tasks. He is concerned about Margaret's low mood, is feeling somewhat tired and burdened himself and is unsure what to do for the best. They agree that Bob will also attend the stress group for his own benefit and to better support Margaret. They also agree a programme whereby Margaret can gradually increase her activity levels. Margaret performs some gentle exercise in Anne's office, conducted as a behavioural experiment to test out the idea that a raised heart rate is not dangerous. Although Margaret remains nervous about over-doing things she begins to feel more confident that increased heart rate does not mean a heart attack is imminent.

It should be noted that, even if the person seems convinced by your advice, he or she is still only likely to believe you are completely right after having personal experience – as Margaret does after the behavioural experiment. This is a reason for using goal-setting (see Chapter 6) – helping people to set small goals that do not arouse too much anxiety for either themselves or their family.

Points for reflection

- Think about two people you have worked with recently. Based on your knowledge of them are you able to describe what their beliefs about illness and disease might be?
- Can you think of any misconceptions you regularly come across with people you care for?
- Below are a series of statements that show what misconceptions people can have. Think about what you might say to them.

  'Any sort of excitement could be bad if you have heart problems.'

  'I have diabetes so I must eat special diabetic foods which are very expensive.'

  'I'm too young for my smoking to have caused chronic lung disease.'

Chronic disease management for long-term conditions

'Arthritis is caused by living somewhere cold and wet and I always have a warm home.'

'I can't have asthma – it only affects children.'

'I can tell when my blood pressure is going up, so that's when I take my tablets. I don't bother the rest of the time.'

Chapter 4
Unhelpful coping behaviour

Learning outcomes

By the end of this chapter you will be able to:

- describe the link between fear and avoidance coping
- discuss an unhelpful pattern of activity with patients.

Introduction

There are many different ways that people cope with their long-term condition, some of which can be very helpful to their prognosis and quality of life. Unfortunately, many people adopt ways of coping that are not helpful.

When people are first diagnosed with a long-term condition they may run through a range of thoughts and emotions. For example, let's consider Karen, a fit young mother of two children who is also a secretary at a local firm.

Case example 8

Karen

Karen has just been told that she has rheumatoid arthritis. Here are a few of the thoughts and feelings that Karen reported.

- 'I was really frightened when they told me. I thought "What have I done to deserve this? It means that I'm old before my time"'
- 'My body is going to change and that scares me – will I end up disfigured and stuck in a wheelchair? Why should my husband stay with a crippled wife? I won't blame him if he

leaves me – it's too much to ask for someone to care for me.'

- 'How am I going to cope with my children? Will I be able to be a proper mum to them?'
- 'I'm probably going to have to give up my job as the arthritis gets worse. How will we afford to live?'
- 'What can I do and what shouldn't I do? I'm frightened that I might make my problem worse if I do too much.'
- 'People are just going to think that I'm lazy when I can't do things.'
- 'I'm really worried about the injections into my knees – how will I cope with the pain?'

(Partly based on work by Edwards *et al.*, 2001)

You can see that Karen's main feelings are fear and anxiety. She is thinking that the worst is going to happen ('I'll end up in a wheelchair and my husband will leave me'). A simple model that has been used to explain the relationship between beliefs and coping in people with chronic pain is the fear–avoidance model (Vlaeyen and Linton, 2000).

Figure 4.1

The fear–avoidance model of chronic pain
(After J.W.S. Vlaeyen and S.J. Linton, PAIN 2000; 85:317–332. Used with permission.)

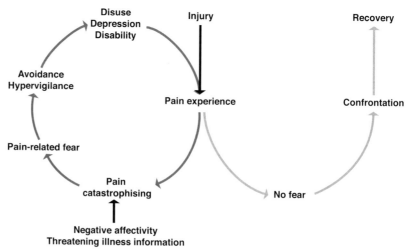

In this model, people fear the worst about their symptoms and what they mean. They then are anxious about situations that may bring their symptoms on or that they believe may make them worse – like

Unhelpful coping behaviour

Steve in Case example 6 and Karen in Case example 8. This can result in them avoiding activities, social withdrawal and lead to more anxiety and depression. In contrast, people who do not fear their symptoms are more likely to cope well with their condition.

Figure 4.2   **Effect of misconceptions on disability**

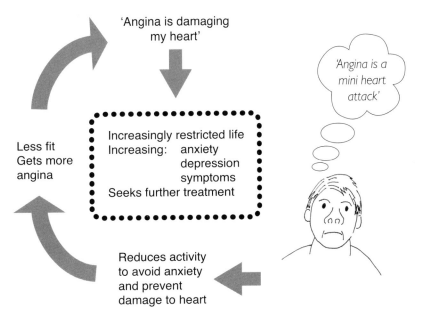

The man in Figure 4.2 is following the left-hand part of Vlaeyan and Linton's model, by fearing his symptoms and avoiding activity, rather like Graham in Chapter 2. In people with chronic back pain, *fear* of pain plays a greater part in the development of disability than the pain itself (Linton and Boersma 2004). Karen is in danger of adopting this model as she is so frightened by her diagnosis. She was already contemplating having to leave work and use a wheelchair.

The woman in Figure 4.3 is more like Omar – she knows that episodes of angina do not do permanent damage to the heart, and so she is following the right-hand part of the fear–avoidance model.

However, it is not simply fear of developing pain or worsening symptoms that contributes to poor coping. Another way that people cope with a long-term condition is by falling into the 'overactivity–rest trap'.

Figure 4.3   **Effect of positive beliefs on disability**

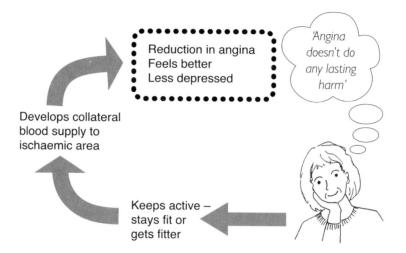

What is the overactivity–rest trap?

Overactivity-rest trap

The overactivity–rest trap was first described in people with chronic back pain, but the same thing happens in other long-term conditions. If you ask a group of people with a long-term condition if their symptoms are constant many will say no, that they come and go. They will say that they have 'good days' and 'bad days'. Case example 9 illustrates what we mean.

Case example 9

Steve and his garden

Let's catch up with Steve (from Case example 6). After his chest infection he and Sally had worked out a plan to help him gradually recover his fitness, and he had stuck to it fairly well for a while. But as time went on he forgot about gradually increasing and then maintaining his activity levels.

Now, six months later, he is getting worried and depressed. It is spring, the garden hasn't been dug properly over the winter and he wants to get his seeds in the ground, so he needs to get down to work. But he is finding it increasingly difficult.

'It's no good,' he said to his wife, 'I felt great at the weekend. I managed to dig a whole section, rake it over and get the cabbage seeds in. I thought I'd be able to do more, but I've felt too tired and poorly the last couple of days. I've had to put my feet up and take it easy, and now it's raining. I'll never get the garden dug.'

'This keeps happening, having a couple of good days and then a week of feeling ill. And I seem to be getting worse. Maybe we should think about moving, I can't manage the garden any more – I'm useless!'

This is a classic description of having 'good' days and 'bad' days. Steve is in the overactivity–rest trap. He has good days followed by days when he feels too tired or ill to do anything. This is because on the good days he does too much and ends up overtired and needs to rest to recover.

It appears to be common sense to wait until you feel well, until your disease 'goes away' for a bit, before doing something that is going to be difficult or tiring. Unfortunately this way of coping is often reinforced when people say 'Listen to your body!', 'Do what you can', 'Pace yourself'.

The result is that many people wait to see how they feel when they wake up each day before deciding if they should do anything active. If they feel good they catch up on jobs that they have had to leave on bad days. The problem with this way of coping is that we lose fitness more quickly than we gain it (Ready *et al.,* 1981). Any gain in fitness from being active on the good days is more than outweighed by the period of resting. People who take more rest become less physically fit – you can see this in Figure 4.4.

Figure 4.4   The overactivity–rest trap

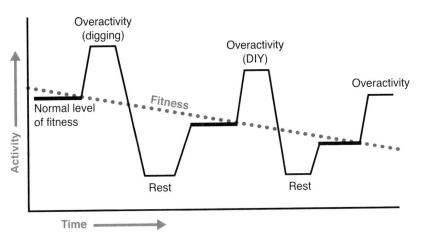

This shows that, while Steve's over-enthusiastic rounds of gardening had the potential to improve his fitness, this was lost because he needed to rest to recover, and his fitness actually reduced.

Why does reduced fitness cause problems?

Muscles that are less fit do not use oxygen as efficiently as fit ones, so that the heart has to work harder to provide them with oxygen and needs more oxygen itself. This is called muscular deconditioning and means that symptoms such as angina or breathlessness in chronic lung disease will come on more quickly as fitness reduces. Figure 4.5 illustrates the physical and psychological effects of deconditioning in people with a long-term condition.

Figure 4.5

The physical and psychological effects of muscular deconditioning

- **Haemodynamic**
  Increased vascular resistance (the heart must work harder to push the blood around)
  Increased resting heart rate (making the heart work harder)

- **Function**
  Decreased exercise tolerance (able to do less before symptoms begin)
  Decreased aerobic fitness
  Decreased balance

- **Musculoskeletal**
  Decreased muscle mass/bulk (less muscle to do the work)
  Decreased strength of bones, cartilage and connective tissue

- **Psychological**
  Decreased well-being (feeling worse)
  Decreased activity scores (believing they can do less)

(After Villani et al., 2000)

The way to reverse the overactivity–rest trap is by goal-setting, which is discussed in detail later in this book. It is a very powerful technique that can help people to get back to doing activities that they have abandoned because of illness.

Points for reflection

- Can you think of someone that you have cared for whose fear of developing symptoms led them to avoid being active?
- Do you hear people talking about good days and bad days? How have you dealt with these conversations in the past?
- Think about how you might suggest this is managed (we will discuss strategies in Chapter 6).

Chapter 5
Overcoming resistance to change

Learning outcomes

By the end of this chapter you will be able to:

- describe the main components of behaviour–change counselling
- understand the importance of self-efficacy in promoting behaviour change
- describe a number of problem-solving techniques to reduce barriers to behaviour change
- give a brief overview of the evidence for this approach.

Introduction

Over the years it has become apparent that telling people to stop risky behaviour is often not enough (Whitehead, 2001). Why is it that some people don't take the advice of health workers?

The stages of change model (SCM)

Stages of change model

Prochaska and DiClemente (1984) proposed a model of change which they called the 'transtheoretical model of behaviour change', but which tends to be referred to as the 'stages of change model' or SCM for short. This model is based on the idea that behaviour change does not happen all at once – it might be easier if it did! Instead people go through different stages as they attempt to change their behaviour. The six stages are:

- **Pre-contemplation**: not thinking about changing their habits.

- **Contemplation:** considering change, but rather ambivalent about it (we discuss this ambivalence in more detail later).

- **Preparation:** deciding they will make a change, and are doing things such as finding out about support groups, or searching the internet for the best way to make the change as easy as possible.

- **Action:** they make a change – but it depends on their will power. This stage is short-lived (up to six months but can also be just a few hours); people either succeed with their action, or they don't. This is when they need most support to try to help them to keep on track.

- **Maintenance/relapse:** people who successfully stay on track are said to be in maintenance – they are on their way to permanent behaviour change. They still need occasional support but they are successfully incorporating the new behaviour into their lives. Relapse is a common part of maintenance – not many people successfully change an entrenched behaviour (such as smoking) without at least one relapse. The biggest danger here is that the relapse causes the individual to give up completely and to revert to their original behaviour pattern.

- **Termination:** The new behaviour is now completely a part of the individual's life, and there is no longer a threat of relapse back to the old risky behaviour.

People will often cycle between the different stages, and may even miss stages out. Although the SCM is often depicted as a wheel, Prochaska *et al.* (1992) later envisaged it as a spiral which people would slide up and down as they negotiated the various stages.

The SCM has been applied to many programmes which attempt to encourage a change in risk behaviours, such as smoking, drinking, or eating the wrong foods. But not all applications of the model are successful. A systematic review of the use of the SCM in health behaviour interventions found that interventions were often not matched to the stage that the study participants were at, and therefore evidence for the efficacy of the model is lacking (Bridle *et al.*, 2005). Further (and better designed) research is required before a stronger statement of efficacy can be made.

Health behaviour change counselling

Changing health behaviour

In this section we introduce key elements of health behaviour change counselling that are helpful for managing long-term conditions. However, it is only an introduction; if health workers wish to use this form of counselling, it is advisable that they seek training from accredited sources.

Take a look at Case example 10 – this is an example of a clinic follow-up visit (the text in the square brackets is what they might be thinking). Do you recognise any aspect of the conversation or the thoughts or feelings that the health worker is having?

Case example 10

Sanjit

Health worker: Hello Sanjit, how have you been?

Sanjit: Fine, everything's going OK. [*I hope she doesn't ask about smoking again.*]

Health worker: Last time I talked to you about your smoking. Have you managed to give up? [*Have you done as you've been told?*]

Sanjit: I've not really managed to get round to that, there's so much happening and I feel so stressed, I don't think that I could give up just yet. [*She doesn't understand my problems.*]

Health worker: I told you that you were more likely to have further problems with your breathing if you continue to smoke. [*This is a waste of my time!*]

Sanjit: Yes, I know, but …

Health worker: (interrupting) Well, you know what you should do; I suggest you seriously think about it before we next meet. [*I've got better things to do than talk to people who don't listen. I knew he would be difficult. You would think that he would really want to give up smoking because of his asthma.*]

Sanjit: Yes I will. [*She's no help. How could I give up smoking with my job? What's the point of me coming here?*]

You can see that this encounter has made things worse, Sanjit feels unsupported and resentful; he is considering not coming for future follow-ups, which may mean that changes in his health will be missed. Look over the conversation above: What is wrong with it? What does the health worker do that makes it worse? What would you change in this consultation?

Resistance and ambivalence

In the conversation above, Sanjit feels he is being asked to do something that he thinks would be difficult or impossible to do. He becomes defensive and shows resistance to the health worker's message. The health worker begins to feel that Sanjit is difficult and sees him as someone who would be resistant to any help. From the start the health worker appears to believe that Sanjit should just do as she says, and doesn't try to see things from his point of view. This lack of understanding and empathy means that Sanjit is more likely to fail to change his behaviour, and be labelled as non-compliant (Shinitzky and Kub, 2001).

An effective encounter between a person and a health worker can remove the barriers to change (Shinitzky and Kub, 2001), but it is very common for the behaviour of the health worker to be the cause of the resistance (Doherty and Roberts, 2002). This is shown by the 'yes... but' reaction of Sanjit. The 'yes... but' scenario happens when a patient gives arguments in defence of the status quo as described by Doherty and Roberts, 2002. Resistance is shown when patients:

- argue
- interrupt or cut-off the interviewer
- deny the problem or blame others, or
- ignore what the health worker is saying by not giving responses or by side-tracking.

Rollnick *et al.* (1997, p. 193) state 'Resistance should be a signal for the health worker to back off and change their approach'.

The health worker in above sums up the feelings of many health workers with the phrase: 'You would think that he would really want to give up smoking because of his asthma.' Miller and Rollnick (2002) give the phrase 'you would think...' as one that captured the frustration of health workers when confronted by resistance to a change in behaviour that could help to save the person's life.

Sanjit is ambivalent about smoking, this means he has mixed feelings (Doherty and Roberts, 2002). He knows that the smoking is harming him, but feels that he can't give it up because it has benefits for him, it helps him cope with stress at work. Most of us have felt ambivalent at some point in our lives, when we both want change and fear it. Ambivalence is a common feeling and a routine part of facing change (Miller and Rollnick, 2002). Problems occur when people become stuck in ambivalence and can't move on. As we saw from the clinic scenario at the beginning of this chapter, trying to push people the way we think they should go does not work.

For people to make changes in their behaviour, they need to see how important it is to make the change, and believe that they can do it. Health behaviour change counselling was developed from motivational interviewing to facilitate this change in busy clinical situations. First we'll look at motivational interviewing and its evidence base.

What is motivational interviewing and how does it work?

Motivational interviewing

Motivational interviewing is defined as 'a client-centred, directive method for enhancing intrinsic motivation to change by exploring and resolving ambivalence' (Miller and Rollnick, 2002, p. 25). So what does that really mean?

Miller and Rollnick emphasise the 'spirit' of motivational interviewing as a way of being with people, and how the way in which you approach the interview process is vital.

Motivational interviewing involves:

- **collaboration** (a partnership between patient and health worker)
- **evocation** (drawing on the patient's own resources and motivation)
- **autonomy** (backing the patient's ability to be self-directed).

This contrasts with traditional forms of patient/professional encounter, where there is often:

- **confrontation** rather than collaboration
- **education** rather than evocation
- **professional authority** rather than patient autonomy.

The methods of motivational interviewing are to:

- work with the **ambivalence** felt by the patient

- increase their feelings of the importance of the change
- increase their belief that they can do it (**self-efficacy**)
- increase their readiness to change without creating **resistance**.

In order to achieve this Miller and Rollnick (2002) have described four guiding principles of motivational interviewing. Bundy (2004) included one more principle (avoid argument), which produces a simple acronym, DEARS:

- **D**evelop discrepancy
- **E**xpress empathy
- **A**void argument
- **R**oll with resistance
- **S**upport self-efficacy

The following text outlines each of these and their importance in motivational interviewing.

Developing discrepancy

Using reflective listening with the client does not mean that they have to accept the way they are, or that they simply off-load all of their problems while the health worker empathises with them. We need to help clients to see what the difference is between the current problem and the ideal situation; this is done by developing discrepancy (Miller and Rollnick, 2002; Bundy, 2004). Goals for behaviour change should come from the client, not the health worker. However, he or she may be ambivalent about changing their behaviour, so they are stuck between wanting to set a goal and not wanting to. By showing (and perhaps increasing) the discrepancy between the present situation and the important goal, the health worker can help the client to overcome ambivalence. Look at the following conversation.

Client: I know that I need to lose weight. I used to be thin when I was younger but it's crept on over the years, I know that I'll never get back to that weight again. I've tried diets before and lost weight for a while, then it's come back on again.

Health worker: So you were happier with your weight when you were younger, but you're unhappy with it now. Are there reasons why you are unhappy with your weight?

Client: Well, apart from the health problems, I'd like to be a bit thinner for my daughter's wedding in six months' time – I've seen a lovely outfit, but the largest size is 18 and I'm a 22.

Health worker: Your daughter is getting married and you'd like to be thinner as you've seen the perfect outfit. That gives you six months to drop a couple of dress sizes. How important is it for you to get into that dress? On a scale of one to ten, where one is not important and ten is very important, where would you say you are?

Client: Well, if you put it like that, I'd say that it's eight.

In this extract, the health worker has helped to increase the discrepancy between the present situation and the desired goal, and found out how important it is to the client. Asking about the importance of the behaviour change is a strategy that will be covered later. Another method of highlighting ambivalence and developing discrepancy is the decisional balance sheet, where the client writes down both the advantages and disadvantages of changing their behaviour, and the advantages and disadvantages of staying the same and not changing thir behaviour. A copy of a decisional balance sheet, which you can give to clients, can be found in Appendix 1.

Expressing empathy

The healthcare professional needs to hear and accept what the client is saying. This doesn't necessarily mean agreeing with everything they say, but being non-judgemental and understanding of the client's viewpoint. This is done by active listening and reflection, where the health worker responds to what the person has told them by paraphrasing back what they have said. Consider the following example.

Client: It's been really difficult to get out for a daily walk. My wife hasn't been well at all, she's been confused and so I can't leave her. The nurses come in every day but they aren't there during the night, so I'm tired out now.

Health worker: It sounds like you've been having a rough time with your wife's ill health and confusion. You're so tired from caring for her during the night and worried about leaving her that you haven't been able to manage your daily walk.

Reflecting back to the person in this way not only shows that the health worker understands why the person hasn't been for a walk, but also empathises with their situation and shows interest.

Avoiding argument

It is counter-productive to argue for a change in behaviour if the person argues against it. The health worker should not impose their viewpoint or their goals as this will provoke the patient to defend their own viewpoint, with the effect of entrenching their opposition to change (Bundy, 2004).

> **Health worker:** You must lose weight. It's making your arthritis worse and that's why your knees are so painful.
>
> **Person:** But I've tried before and dieting has never worked. I don't eat very much as it is, and I never eat fatty food. My mother was a big woman and I think that I've just inherited her genes. She couldn't lose weight either.

The imposition of a goal on the person above has caused her to argue with the health worker. As Bundy (2004) says, the goal of motivational interviewing is to 'encourage the patient to hear themselves say why they want to change' (p. 46). If they are provoked into defending their viewpoint, they are actually practising arguments against change, which increases their resistance to change.

Rolling with resistance

The solutions to problems need to be owned and found by the client. When you start to see resistance, that's when the health worker needs to 'roll with the resistance'. Doherty and Roberts (2002) suggest a variety of strategies that are particularly useful in the early stages of the professional–patient relationship when there is a greater likelihood of resistance. These include:

- using reflections rather than closed questions. (this avoids the 'yes...but' scenario)
- letting the clients give all their reasons (without interruption) for not being able to make a particular behaviour change
- highlighting ambivalence

- suspending advice-giving – tempting as it might be!

Below we give you a scenario that illustrates the points made above. These are shown in italics.

Client: I couldn't stop smoking, so it's pointless talking to me about it. I know that I should stop, and I'd like to, but you people just don't understand how hard it is. You don't know what it's like to be out of work and stuck at home all day with an elderly mother. You don't know how stressed I am. I need to keep smoking to cope; otherwise I'd go out of my mind. [*This person is showing resistance to change. The health worker is letting the person list all of their reasons for not changing.*]

Health worker: You're right; even if I was still a smoker, I wouldn't know how hard it was for you to stop and I don't know what it's like for you to be stuck at home all day with your mother. [*This is an example of reflection.*]

So I'm not going to tell you to stop smoking. However it would help me to understand if you would tell me what it's like for you. [*The health worker has suspended advice-giving.*]

On the one hand, you've told me that you'd like to stop smoking but on the other, it helps you with to cope with the stress of being unemployed and living with your elderly mother. [*Ambivalence is being highlighted here.*]

Support self-efficacy

Before we go into detail about this in relation to motivational interviewing it is important to have a little knowledge of what is meant by self-efficacy.

Self-efficacy is how confident you are in your ability to succeed in achieving a goal. This can be very situation-specific. For example, you may feel confident in reading a map but lack confidence about assembling a flat-packed cupboard. You may feel confident that you could give up eating french fries but not confident that you could exercise for an hour a day.

Research has shown that the more you believe in your ability to succeed at a particular task, the more likely you are to succeed. Of course this may be because we already have a pretty good idea of our own ability, but it may also be because if we take on a goal convinced we will fail, This affects our effort and motivation, making failure a self-fulfilling prophecy.

An American psychologist, Albert Bandura (1994), describes four main ways in which we develop self-efficacy:

- **mastery:** previous experience of success is the strongest way to build belief about future success. The opposite is also true, repeated failure is the best way to reduce confidence.

- **vicarious experience:** seeing someone else succeed at a task can help us to believe that we would succeed too. This effect is stronger the more we see ourselves as similar to the person we've observed. Again this also works the other way, seeing someone like us fail can make us believe that we would also fail.

- **social persuasion:** encouragement can undoubtedly help people try harder and keep on trying. It has to be used carefully though – if the person you've encouraged believes that their success depended on you then this lowers their own feeling of self-efficacy. Even worse, if you encourage a person to take on something that defeats them you will lower their self-efficacy. As Bandura says, people who are successful at using social persuasion to boost another person's self-efficacy do so by encouraging people to set goals that will end in success.

- **feedback**; this is from the person's own body and emotions. People also take account of messages from their body when they think about their possibility of success. If someone feels too weak or very anxious when they think about a task they will be less confident that they will succeed.

All of this suggests that if we can bolster people's feelings of self-efficacy for the tasks that they face (losing weight, taking more exercise, changing their diet, etc.) they will be more likely to succeed.

So what are the rules for self-efficacy?

- Set small achievable goals that the client is likely to succeed at and which they themselves feel they are very likely to succeed with. You may regard the goal as being well below the person's ability, or set so low that it will make no difference to their health, but this is not the point. If the person feels that the goal is very difficult they will be much less likely to attempt it, or if they do make an attempt they are more likely to fail. If they succeed at a first few small goals they are more likely to continue to build on this and eventually achieve a change that does improve their health.

- Use vicarious experience, giving examples of other people, who are like the person, who have tried and succeeded. Obviously you can't break confidentiality and give names but it can help to tell anecdotes such as 'I had another gentleman who is a farmer like you. He did very well. He started by walking around one of his fields twice each day; now he goes on long distance tramping trails for a week at a time!'

- Use persuasion but make it realistic and slowly fade it out once the person is beginning to gain confidence.

- Never set goals that make the person nervous or for which they feel they don't have the strength.

From this we can see that self-efficacy is a good predictor of whether the person will be successful with their behaviour change (Miller and Rollnick, 2002). The person may believe that it is very important to make a change, but also believe that it would be impossible for them to achieve this, making it more likely that they will not make sufficient effort.

It is also important for the health worker to believe that the person will be successful. If they don't believe that the change can be achieved then the person may pick up on this, which can cause demotivation (Miller and Rollnick, 2002).

> **Client:** I've had a bad week with my diet, I've put two pounds on.
>
> **Health worker:** You've been doing really well and you've lost over a stone in weight; that's fantastic. You've shown how motivated you are. What was different about last week?
>
> **Client:** I just wanted to eat more, I was fed up with the diet.
>
> **Health worker:** What do you think you would need to do in the next week to get back on track?

In this scenario the health worker asks the person to identify the reason for the lapse, and also to solve the problem. This is one of the main features of problem solving, that, whenever possible, the person should develop the solutions themselves. Where the person can't think of a solution the health worker should not immediately jump in with advice but should ask the person's permission to suggest some potential solutions that they may then choose from.

> **Client:** I don't know what to do.
>
> **Health worker:** Well, I know some things that other people have found helpful. Would you like me to run through them?

The evidence for motivational interviewing

Motivational interviewing was developed for use with people with alcohol addiction, and the majority of the evidence for its efficacy comes from substance abuse literature. A meta-analysis of controlled trials of motivational interviewing was published by Burke *et al.* (2003). Of 30 trials included in the analysis, 19 targeted substance abuse, 4 targeted diet and exercise, 2 smoking and the rest were related to HIV risk behaviour, treatment adherence and eating disorders. The meta-analysis found that motivational interviewing was significantly more effective than no treatment or placebo for alcohol and drug abuse, and diet and exercise problems, but not for smoking or HIV risk behaviour. Motivational interviewing was equivalent to other active psychotherapeutic treatments for alcohol or drug abuse (Burke *et al.,* 2003).

Studies that have reported after the meta-analysis continue to show similar evidence for the use of motivational interviewing in behaviour change for risk reduction. Interventions aimed at changing diet tend to report positive findings (for example, Bowen *et al.,* 2002; Elliot *et al.,* 2004; Resnicow *et al.,* 2002) while those that report smoking cessation have more equivocal results, with negative findings (for example, Ershoff *et al.,* 2001; Smith *et al.,* 2001; Stotts *et al.,* 2002; Wakefield *et al.,* 2004) outnumbering the positive ones (for example, Cigrang *et al.,* 2002; Emmons *et al.,* 2001). It should be noted that, as motivational interviewing is a fairly new intervention, the evidence base is changing constantly, and people who wish to ensure that they use evidence-based methods should be encouraged to keep in touch with the literature (McCambridge, 2004).

Health behaviour change counselling

Motivational interviewing is acknowledged to be time intensive, however, Rollnick *et al.*, (1997) devised a brief version of motivational interviewing for use in busy clinical situations: health behaviour change counselling.

Health behaviour change counselling has three phases:

1. quick assessment

2. problem identification

3. target and follow-up.

The following advice is adapted from Rollnick *et al.* (1997, p. 197).

Phase 1 – Quick assessment

The main aim of this phase is to build rapport with the person, and then to assess motivation for the behaviour change, and self-confidence in being able to succeed.

- Rapport is established by asking non-judgemental, open questions about the behaviour change.

- Motivation is established by assessing how much the person wants to change their risk behaviour by asking about how motivated they feel about the behaviour change on a scale of one to ten, where one is not motivated and ten is very motivated. If motivation is seven or more then this is OK. You can ask about confidence. If motivation is less than seven then try to increase this.

  Another way to increase motivation is to ask the person for the pros and cons of the risk behaviour, for example: 'What do you like about smoking?' or 'What do you dislike about smoking?'. Summarise the points for the person and then ask, 'Where does that leave you?'.

- Confidence is assessed in a similar way by asking how confident the person is that they will succeed, if one is not confident, and ten is very confident. Again, a score of seven or more means that the person is likely to be confident enough to succeed. If the person is not confident (and it is possible for someone to have high motivation and low confidence) then try to identify strategies to increase confidence (see below).

Phase 2 – Patient identifies problems and solutions

There are some questions that you can ask in order to help the person to identify the problems, and to find solutions to increase motivation and confidence. For example:

- 'Why are you at [number less than seven] and not one?' Asking this type of scaling question helps to get the person to identify arguments for change which can increase motivation.

- 'What would need to happen for you to move from [number less than seven] to eight or nine?'

You could use different strategies such as detailing the pros and cons, or offering non-judgemental information about personal risk. A range of strategies will be discussed in more detail in the section on problem solving. Below is an example of a conversation between a person with a long-term condition and their health worker; the strategies being adopted by the health worker are shown in italics.

Health worker: I guess you may be a little fed-up of people telling you to diet. I'm not going to do that, but it would help me if you could tell me a little about the sort of things that you eat on an average day. *[Establishing rapport]*

Client: Well, I try to eat properly. I'll start the day OK, but then I get bored in the evening and start to look for things to snack on while I'm watching TV. I know that doing this isn't helping with my weight problem, but I can't seem to get out of the habit. I've tried lots of times, and I try not to buy things that are fatty, but I give in to temptation. *[Person lists problems without interruption]*

Health worker: Although you try to eat properly, you've got into the habit of snacking in the evening while watching TV. How do you feel about your weight? *[Continuing to establish rapport]*

Person: Sometimes I feel OK, but if I see myself in the mirror I feel bad. I think 'Oh my goodness, who is that fat woman?'. It makes me feel down when I realise that the fat woman is me. I can't get any nice clothes to fit, and I don't like going into the shops to try them on. It's difficult.

Health worker: So, when you can't see yourself you feel OK, but you feel down when you catch sight of yourself in the mirror, and it's difficult to get nice clothes. *[Highlighting ambivalence and developing discrepancy]*

Client: Yes, and I'd really like my husband to be proud of me. He says that he's OK about the way I am, but I'd like to look good for him as well as for myself.

Health worker: You think your husband is OK about how you are now, but you think he would be proud of you if you lost weight, and you would be proud of yourself. How about your motivation? On a scale of one to ten, if one is not motivated and ten is very motivated, how motivated are you to lose weight? *[Developing discrepancy, assessing motivation]*

Client: I'd say about a seven.

Health worker: Why are you a seven and not a one? *[Scaling question]*

Client: I'm not a one, because I do have motivation, I realise that I can't go on being this weight – it's affecting my health. *[Identification of reasons to change]*

Health worker: If you did decide to try to lose weight, how confident are you that you'll succeed, if one is not confident and ten is very confident? *[Assessing confidence]*

Client: I think that I'd be a four.

Health worker: What would need to happen to move your confidence to say an eight or nine? *[Identifying possible solutions]*

Client: I'm not sure. Maybe if I felt that people were supporting me, helping me over the bad times. And maybe if my husband and I didn't watch so much TV in the evening, that might help. *[Developing strategies to increase confidence]*

Health worker: Is there anything I can do to help to increase your confidence that you will succeed? *[If no ideas, offer possible strategies]*

Client: I don't know. Would you be prepared to see me once a week and weigh me? Maybe knowing that you'd do that would help me to be more confident that this time I could do it. *[Identification of a strategy by the person to increase confidence]*

Phase 3 – Target and follow-up

If the person is willing to try to change, the next step is to set small, manageable goals. Remember that it is very important for the patient to have success early in the programme, as this will reinforce the behaviour, motivate them and increase their self-efficacy.

If people are not ready to do try to change and don't want to do anything, then it is important to leave them feeling that they can start later.

> **Client:** I'm not sure that I can cope with all of this right at the moment. I'm finding it a bit difficult to come to terms with what's happening.
>
> **Health worker:** That's fine. You don't have to do anything that you are not ready for. Is there anything that I can do to help you?
>
> **Client:** No, I can't think of anything at the moment.
>
> **Health worker:** You know that I'm here if you need to talk things over, just phone me. Is it OK if I raise these topics with you next time we talk?
>
> **Client:** Yes, that would be good.
>
> **Health worker:** [*summarising*] Today, we've talked about the things that the doctor had told you and about some of the issues he raised. At the moment, you don't feel that you can make any changes, but you know that you can call me if you want any help. You've got your copy of the information we recommend, so that you can look through that over the next week, and as part of this programme you will come back to clinic to see me next Thursday at 2pm. See you then.

Problem solving

Problem solving

As we said earlier, if the solutions come from the client then they are more likely to use them. But that doesn't mean that you can't help. Problem solving (D'Zurilla and Goldfried, 1971) is a strategy that has four steps:

1. Problem identification: identify the specific problem that is preventing the person from changing their behaviour. For example, 'I can't lose weight' is very broad; ask: 'Why do you think that is?'. This could include specific times or reasons for the person to feel that they will fail. 'My mother keeps baking cakes and would be upset if I didn't eat them, that's why I'm fat.'

2. **Solution generation:** these should come from the person. There are different strategies that you can use to help the person to come up with ideas. These include:

- *Brain-storming* to find a list of possible solutions. Allow all of the possible solutions to come forward without judging them; sometimes a solution that may appear silly can lead to success for that person or trigger off another better idea.

- Drawing up a list of the *costs and benefits* of each solution. This will help to spot any potential problems and to generate solutions to overcome that problem.

- *What could work?* Ask the person about past successes, or whether they know of ideas other people have used to succeed.

3. **Selecting one solution to test:** once there is a list of possible solutions, the person can decide which they would like to try. If they are unsure, then they can review the costs and benefits (see above) to work out which solution would suit them best. They can then, with your help, plan how they are going to introduce this solution into their daily life.

4. **Evaluating the outcome of the behaviour change:** if the person has been successful, they should be asked to list the improvements that they have experienced. This will help with motivation and maintenance. If there have been setbacks or failures it can help to ask the person 'What have you learned from this attempt?'. Producing something positive from the failure may help to prevent the person from punishing themselves and possibly slipping back into other risky behaviours that they have been able to change.

Rollnick *et al.* (1997) suggested the following main points:

- If at all possible the solutions should come from the person.

- Do not offer simple, single solutions – there is always more than one way to do something.

- Only supplement with your ideas when the person has given all of theirs, and then only if permission has been given or the person asks for advice.

- Encourage people to solve one problem at a time. People often have multiple problems. Trying to change too much at once is far more likely to fail. If the person is motivated to change but not sure where to start, then use a 'triage' style. This means considering:

1. which is the most important change to make
2. which change has the greatest chance of success, and
3. which change would give the earliest success.

Sometimes the most important change has the least chance of success at that time, so it may be better to choose a goal that would give an early success. Doing this is reinforcing and can boost motivation and confidence.

Points for reflection

- Think about some of your own recent consultations with people. On reflection can you see where someone may have been resisting?

- What kind of verbal and body language did you notice? If you noticed this now during a consultation, would you manage it differently? Think about how.

- Four principles of motivational interviewing were discussed. Consider how you could incorporate these into a discussion with someone.

- Consider the principles of problem solving. Think about some questions or prompts that you might be able to use in your work to encourage people to identify their own solutions.

Chapter 6
Goal setting to change behaviour

Learning outcomes

At the end of this chapter you will be able to:

- understand why goal setting is important
- describe the principles of goal setting
- give examples of common setbacks and what to do about them.

Introduction

Goal setting is one of the most important skills in helping people change. It is the best way to reverse the overactivity–rest trap as well as to increase activity levels safely, in a way that is likely to become a lifelong habit.

This simple, but very powerful, technique was first theorised by Edwin Locke in the 1960s. He defined a goal as 'the object or aim of an action' (Locke and Latham, 2002, p. 705). Interestingly he found that people were motivated to try harder to achieve a goal that was moderately difficult compared with one that was either very easy or very hard (Locke and Latham, 2002). We know that goal setting is the best and simplest way to increase self-efficacy (Locke & Latham, 2002).

Goals must be what the individual person wants to achieve. *Resistance or ambivalence* can be overcome using motivational interviewing techniques. You are there to:

1. get the person started
2. supply *motivation,* and
3. support them until they learn the technique of goal setting for themselves.

Chronic disease management for long-term conditions

People must choose the goals and decide the point at which they feel they have mastered that goal and are ready to move on to a harder one. If you simply give them a goal, or force them to step it up before they feel they have mastered that level, it is much less likely that they will carry it out or that it will become a permanent change in their behaviour.

Goals, targets and baselines

Goals, targets and baselines

- The *goal* is what the person wishes to achieve: get back to work, lose 20 lb, stop smoking, eat five pieces of fruit or vegetables a day, be able to walk five miles, get back to playing golf.
- The *target* is the short-term goal that you set with the person on the way to the goal.
- The *baseline* is the starting level at the beginning of the goal setting.

Do it SMARTER

Use the acronym **SMARTER**. Goals and targets should be:

- *specific*: clearly defined. 'I'm going to exercise more' is a poor goal; 'I'm going to go for a 30 minute walk everyday in my lunch hour' is excellent.
- *measurable*: 'I'm going to get back to gardening' is bad; what does it mean – cutting the grass once a month or opening a market garden? 'I want to be able to do all my own gardening' is a better goal, but not specific enough for a target. 'I'm going to do 20 minutes gardening five times a week' is a good target; it is measurable and gives reinforcement every time the patient ticks it off on their goal sheet.
- *achievable*: nothing is less helpful than failing a target or a goal.
- *realistic*: 'I'm going to lose 3 stone in the next 2 months' is unrealistic and will almost definitely be failed, which is punishing and lowers self-efficacy. 'I'm going to lose one lb a week' is more realistic, and if it is exceeded is even more reinforcing.

- *time bound*: goals are much more likely to be carried out if a specific time is set. 'I'll do a walk just before my lunch every day' is a better goal than 'I'll take a walk each day.' Putting a time to goals and taking medication has been shown to improve compliance.

- *efficacy scored*: ask, for each goal, how confident the client is that he or she will succeed. If it is seven or less ask them to make it slightly easier so that it would be an eight out of ten.

- *rewarding*: goals that are not rewarding will not motivate the person or lead to the establishment of a new health behaviour.

More tips

Having a diary is a great way to record the goals and if possible the person should be the one to write down the goals in the diary. This process will help them to own the goal and is part of the technique of fading so that the person takes over the goal setting. We've included an example of a goal-setting diary in Appendix 4.

Sometimes it is rewarding for the client if their family or carer is involved and gives them praise each time they do the goal. This should only happen if the client says they are happy for another person to be part of the process of goal setting. Indeed partners could also have a diary and set health improvement goals of their own.

If someone has a lot of goals, it is far better to choose just a couple to tackle at first – it helps to keep their motivation for change focused.

If the client has been ill for a long time they may have given up seeking pleasure, going to the cinema, visiting friends, going to the pub. It is therefore very helpful to set goals for these social and enjoyable events, not just for risk factors and health behaviour change.

Any misconceptions of either the client or friends and relatives should be addressed as these could get in the way of achieving the goals. It is important that 'other important people' in the person's life are on board with the goal, otherwise they may not see the importance and may sabotage the programme – 'Do you really have to do that now? I want you to help me with dinner' or 'Are you sure that it's safe to do that? I think you should sit down and rest – that would do you a lot more good'.

Finding the goals

**Finding
the goals**

There are health goals that are likely to be important for the person to achieve, for example, giving up smoking, but there are also personal goals. It is important to consider both, as the aim is to help clients get back to as full and enjoyable a life as possible.

Sometimes you will come across a client who can't think of any hobbies or enjoyable pastimes. It is worth spending some time brainstorming to find things they might like to try or that they did in the dim and distant past when they had more time on their hands. It doesn't need to be active, though of course this is an added bonus; making model boats, stamp collecting, photography, all these will help the patient avoid anxiety and depression and cope with the stress of living with a long-term condition.

The health goals all work together. For example dietary change, exercise and weight loss can all contribute to lowering blood pressure. It is important to emphasise this fact, that each of the goals will help with the others, as you go through setting goals to reduce the risk factors.

A walking programme

One excellent way of increasing physical fitness is a walking programme. In people with heart disease this has been shown to be as effective as a hospital-based programme in increasing physical fitness (Bell, 1998).

This is great exercise for everybody and is free and is more likely to become a lifetime habit than gym work. The walking pace should be brisk enough to cause breathing to speed up a little – mild breathlessness, but the person should still be able to hold a conversation. If they cannot speak easily while walking they need to slow the pace down a little; if they don't feel their breathing quicken at all, they need to speed up the pace.

Even very disabled people should set a walking target. Short distances, even a few hundred yards, or once round the garden, to the first lamp post in the street and back have led to people being able to walk several miles. You should aim to get the person up to two 15-minute, brisk walks a day. If you can build in a reward to the daily walk, for example buying a paper or stopping for a coffee along the way, so much the better.

Relaxation

Relaxation is equally important and a goal can be encouraged that supports finding time for relaxation each day. Any resistance to any of these can be explored using the motivational interviewing techniques described earlier.

Medications

Some people have very complicated medical regimens and can often get confused which to take when and result in poor compliance. This can be helped by setting the various medications as time-bound goals in their diary.

Choosing the targets

Choosing the targets

Once the goals have been found the next step is to break each down into a set of realistic targets. Most lifestyle changes, such as changing diet, are best done in steps and you may need to use problem solving to generate solutions. For example, if the client does not like fruit and vegetables you may have to find those which they have least aversion to (most people like bananas, grapes, potatoes, vine tomatoes, etc.). You may also have to suggest some work-arounds, e.g. having a fruit juice as one portion, or adding apple to a breakfast cereal, as well as ways of incorporating vegetables that are less challenging for the person: leeks in potato mash for example. If the first target is simply the addition of one extra piece of fruit and one portion of vegetable a day, that is probably enough.

Always check the client's self-efficacy (confidence) out of ten – 'How confident are you, out of ten if ten is completely confident, that you will be able to add one piece of fruit and one vegetable to your daily diet?'. Answers of seven or less suggest you should reduce the target, or find another solution through problem solving. Finally, where diet is concerned it is very important to ask who does the cooking, and who buys the food and to get that person involved in the goal setting. If they too are overweight then setting targets with them may also be helpful.

The one exception to the rule of small stages is smoking. It is generally agreed that it is better to go for abstinence and to reinforce continuing abstinence when necessary, helping clients-manage relapses by encouraging them not to 'give up giving up'. 'You can only fail to stop smoking, if you stop quitting' is a phrase some people will connect with. *Ensure that all options to support smoking cessation are explored, for example attendance at a smoking cessation group and prescription of nicotine replacement therapy.* The main thing is to check at each contact if the person is still abstinent and to massively reward continued abstinence, and deal with relapses by offering other solutions from the menu.

Some goals – getting back to playing a whole round of golf, for example – will require the ability to walk for a couple of miles carrying a heavy club bag and driving the ball many times. This may have to be tackled as several separate targets, building up the walking should be happening, but adding the carrying of a shoulder bag, or walking part of the actual course with a half empty bag and using a driving range to build up the strength in the arms may be useful sub-goals. Similarly, with jobs such as decorating, if a person says that they want to redecorate a room you will have to break this down into the various tasks – stripping the old wallpaper for so many minutes each day, sanding woodwork for so many minutes a day, painting and so on. Gardening covers many activities with different levels of intensity of activity.

Setting the right level for a target

By now you will realise the importance of setting the target at the right level. Too easy is not rewarding or motivating, too hard is unlikely to be successful and therefore reduces self-efficacy, motivation and compliance. This is made more complicated because some people will want to impress you by setting very difficult goals; others will be naturally impatient or believe the adage 'no pain, no gain'. These people are at risk of setting goals that are unsustainable and may end in the over-activity–rest trap.

There will also be people who are scared and set goals that are very low. This is not a problem because if they practise every day they will become more confident and these people often go on to make very good progress.

The best place to start with every client is what they do now. When asking someone about their walking, it is more helpful to ask 'How long can you walk for, on the level, without getting symptoms, even on a bad day'. This format gets around a couple of problems. Many people cannot estimate distance accurately, but do know how long they can do something for. Asking about what they can do on a bad day ensures that they are giving an amount that does not produce symptoms. In order to reduce the possibility of someone overestimating what they can do before they get symptoms it is a simple practice to set a target at 80 per cent of what they have said that they can do as the baseline. So, if someone says the longest they can walk for at present is 10 minutes then setting a goal of walking for 30 minutes is likely to be a problem. It would be better to set a goal of no more than 8 minutes for each walk, but perhaps to ask them if they could do this twice a day. If the person practises at this level for a few days or a week, this baseline level of activity can then be reviewed.

Reviewing success and resetting targets

At each meeting all of the goals and targets should be reviewed. Look at each one in the diary and reinforce each example of success. Unless you do this the person will lose interest in self-recording, which is an important part of the process.

Let's have a look at an example of a worked diary, using the template that we have included in Appendix 4. Remember Case examples 6 and 9 – Steve and his garden? What happened to him? Let's catch up.

Case example 11

Steve wins through

Steve went for a check up with his practice nurse, Peter, and told him about his problems with tiredness and reduced fitness. Peter talked to John about the overactivity–rest cycle, and the importance of slowly improving his fitness by not overdoing things. He and Steve then talked through what Steve would like to achieve. This is what Steve recorded as his main goals in the diary:

This week's targets	My target score
1. Mow front lawn on Tuesday and back lawn on Thursday afternoon	7

2. 10 minutes of digging on Monday, Wednesday, Friday afternoon	7
3. 10 minutes of weeding every morning	9
4. Daily walk to get newspaper - 20 minutes	8
5. Shopping with wife Saturday morning	7
6. Take grandchildren to park Sunday afternoon	7

You can see that Steve has been very precise on how much gardening he will do this week, with heavy activities (mowing the lawn and digging) paced out over the week. He has also included other activities that are part of getting fit (walking) and social activities that may contribute to tiredness (shopping and playing with grandchildren) and so did not include gardening targets for those days. Steve visited Peter a couple of weeks later – this is what he said about goal setting:

Peter: Well, how has it gone, Steve?

Steve: I've been really surprised. I didn't think that something so simple would work. I thought that we had set the targets too small. I mean, who would do ten minutes of digging and think that it would get them anywhere? But it has been great. I've actually done more these past two weeks than I've achieved in a month. It's amazing how much you can do when it's spread out over a few days. The garden is starting to take shape, and what's great is that I've had plenty of energy to play with the grandchildren on Sundays, when before I was always too tired. My wife has now started to use a goal diary because she's got arthritis as you know, and when she saw how it helped me to achieve what I wanted to do, well she thought it might help her.

Dealing with problems and setbacks

Let's consider five common problems

- **Falling back into the overactivity–rest trap** because they have been varying the amount of exercise according to how they feel. The person may report: 'You know I said I would walk a

Problems and setbacks

mile, well on Thursday I walked five!'. Your response should be something like 'Well done for walking but my question would be how did you feel on Friday and were you able to achieve Friday's goal?'.

'No – I wasn't able to walk on Friday – I was a bit jiggered! But the five miles will have done me good – won't it?'

'Do you remember me telling you about the overactivity–rest trap? It sounds like you fell into it; you did what you felt like, not what you'd planned.'

- **Raising the targets too quickly**. This can be a particular problem once the person starts to become more confident. It is important to ensure the goals are realistic and achievable.

- **Being ill**. When the person has been ill and unable to do their activities, they need to take the level of activity back a bit. They will have lost a little fitness and would struggle to start back where they left off. They should reset their targets so that they do not have to try too hard.

- **Going on holiday**. If the holiday has been a two-week relaxing break on the beach, then fitness levels may have fallen. The person may need to reduce their target level so that it is not too hard. Sometimes the holiday is an active one in a different part of the country. This is fine, but the person needs to ensure that they don't suddenly try to do too much. A walk length that is easy at home may be more difficult if the holiday area is hillier, so they may need to reduce the length of time walking to account for the greater effort that the walk takes.

- **Competing**. Some people can't help but compete with themselves or others – they must always try to beat their best time or do better than other patients. Competing can end up with people back in the overactivity–rest trap, as they overdo it and so need to rest to recover. When helping to set targets, or when following up on progress with goal setting, remind people to be aware of the problems that competing can bring.

Precautions

When a person tells you that they feel tired or are struggling with their targets, you will need to help them to work out what is wrong. First, check if it is because they are doing more because of a change in routine (having visitors, busy social life, etc.) or whether they are more stressed and not sleeping well (financial problems, family problems, bereavement).

Points for reflection

- Reflect on your approach to setting goals – do you? And if you do, who owns the goals?
- Think about how you could use goal setting with a person you have been having difficulty in motivating.
- Remember SMARTER. How would you use this as part of the process?
- Consider how you might manage a conversation with someone starting out using the goal-setting approach.

Chapter 7
Reducing stress

Learning outcomes

By the end of this chapter you will be able to:

- describe relaxation and the barriers to its success
- guide patients through an exercise to reduce tension
- understand the importance of breathing retraining
- guide patients to use general breathing control to reduce anxiety.

Introduction

Being diagnosed with a long-term illness can be very stressful, both for the person diagnosed and for their family and close friends. Why do people need to learn to relax? Surely it would be enough just to put your feet up at the end of the day and watch TV. This sounds fine, but it is not very helpful when faced with a stressful situation that needs dealing with. How do you prevent the stress from becoming overwhelming? We look more at coping with anxiety and depression in a later chapter. This chapter is about using two different but complementary techniques to reduce the feelings and effects of stress.

What is relaxation?

Relaxation

The way in which relaxation acts on the autonomic nervous system remains unknown, but the fact that it does and that it produces very real physiological changes is obvious to anyone who has learnt the technique.

Feelings that are related to a deeply relaxed state include:

- warm hands and feet, the result of relaxed tone in peripheral blood vessels increasing blood flow to those parts
- a feeling of lethargy and unwillingness to act or move, similar to the feeling just before slipping into sleep
- a warm comfortable state of contentment and security
- increased saliva production
- a complete lack of muscle tension
- a feeling of sinking into the chair or bed, or the opposite, a feeling of floating above it.

If the person reports these feelings you can be fairly certain that they are managing to relax properly. The aim is to teach the person how to achieve this state at any time – not just when listening to a relaxation CD. There are many relaxation programmes available on CD or video, or you may advise people to join a yoga programme. These will be necessary for learning general relaxation. However, it is rapid relaxation formats that are most useful in stressful situations. To help you to understand what these may involve, we have included a transcript of a form of rapid relaxation – tension spotting.

The relaxation programme should move from practising lying down in a warm, quiet room to learning relaxation in a chair to checking for tension throughout the day and relaxing at those times to become a generally more relaxed person.

Regular practice

It is important that the person practices once or twice a day, every day. Obviously you can't force anyone to take it on but you may be able to use motivational interviewing techniques to explore why a person is reluctant if they are.

Resistance to this can come from a feeling that it is a bit 'hippy', or fears that it is like hypnosis and involves handing over control; occasionally you may come across someone who has religious objections. Most commonly the problem is an undefined belief that it is unexplained or explored. It may be worth telling doubters that most of the world's top sports people have a sports psychologist who teaches them to use relaxation to operate at the optimal level.

Our experience of many years of teaching people using relaxation tapes is that around 50 per cent will take to it almost immediately and carry on using it for at least a year, a further 20–30 per cent will struggle at first but begin to appreciate it after a few weeks, and the rest will remain unimpressed, possibly because although they say that they are practising they are not, or they are part of a group who have extreme difficulty in ever relaxing, even with intensive face-to-face training.

Safety notices

It is a good idea to run through the following suggestions and precautions when introducing relaxation:

- Choose a time and place when you won't be disturbed.
- The room should be warm and quiet.
- Ask others to leave you in peace for the 20 minutes you need.
- Don't practise with others because you are likely to keep wondering how they are getting on.
- To start with don't practise where if you fell asleep you might fall over, for example in an upright chair with no arms.
- Don't listen when driving.
- At the end of the relaxation take a moment or two before you stand up or you may become dizzy and fall.

Script for Rapid relaxation:
How to spot tension building up

Tension can often build up gradually in your body throughout the day without you really being aware of it. By taking five minutes to check how you feel and then making some adjustments using your breathing to help you, you can begin to create a more relaxed state at all times, increasing your sense of well being generally.

At any time during your day, tell yourself to be completely still, to 'freeze'. You may be at your desk, standing at the kitchen sink, waiting in a queue, getting dressed, watching television – whatever you choose.

So, be completely still now. Hold your posture for a brief moment or two, but don't hold your breath – keep breathing comfortably and normally.

Now scan through the whole length of your body in your mind's eye – don't alter your posture at all yet, stay still and just as you are, but scan through and see if you can feel any places where you find tension. Remember where these places are as you take a comfortably long breath in now and, as you sigh the breath out, allow your whole body to soften, to 'unfreeze'.

Take a few more breaths like this, a comfortably long breath in, preferably through your nose if you can, and then softly sigh the breath out and feel your body release and let go a little more.

Good. Can you remember where you felt those areas of tension in your body a moment ago? Consciously soften and relax those places more and more as you softly sigh each breath out, nice and gently, gradually releasing a little bit more, relaxing and letting go.

Make little adjustments to your body where you feel they will help – perhaps become more upright in your posture, maybe relaxing your shoulders down away from your ears, releasing your jaw and bringing a hint of a smile to your face – smiling is the nicest way to relax the muscles of your face and jaw – it smooths away any frowns and makes you feel good, too!

With normal comfortable breathing now, in and out through your nose if you can, feel your body releasing tension a little further with each exhalation, releasing from the top of your head, through the whole length of your body, right down to the soles of your feet, a sense of letting go of tension through the whole of your body with each out breath.

Notice any changes that may be occurring. Repeat the process, fine tune your awareness of how your body feels, scanning through the whole length of your body in your mind's eye, releasing and letting go more and more with each out breath.

Bring your attention close to your breathing now and notice how it is. Is it smooth and even or still a bit restless? Don't force or strain your breathing at all and don't worry if it still feels a bit uneven, it will settle into a natural and relaxed rhythm with practice. Just observe how it is now and focus on the rhythm of your breath, gradually moving towards comfortable, easy breathing.

And how do you feel now? How does your physical body feel? Has your mood changed at all?

Observe how you feel in every respect, make a mental note of any changes – your body, your breathing, your mind, your whole being – and then carry on with whatever you were doing previously– until the next time you take five minutes to be still and 'freeze'.

Difficulties in learning to relax

There are four main problems people encounter when learning to relax and people should be warned of these in advance.

● **Wandering mind**: this can lead to annoyance with themselves resulting in frustration rather than relaxation. Assure the person that everyone's mind wanders while listening to the tape or CD, nothing is lost, just bring your mind back to the taped voice and carry on from there.

● **Expecting something more and worrying that it is 'not working'**: relaxation is not an altered state of mind, most of us have experienced the feeling before, lying half asleep in a warm bath, lying on a warm beach, snug in a warm bed just before slipping into sleep. The thing that is new is being able to get that feeling at will.

● **Not practising**: in research in which the tape player secretly recorded how many times the tape had been played it showed that the majority of people who failed to learn had not been practising.

● **Falling asleep**: this is not really a problem unless it happens within the first few minutes of listening so that the person never hears all of the instructions. Indeed many people are pleased because they interpret it as success. Practising in a recliner type chair at a time when they are most alert and not closing the eyes may help them to hear to the end of the tape so that they can memorise the method.

Rare problems

A very small number of people may experience other problems including:

- **Unwanted and unpleasant memories**: If this is persistent then using meditation may be a better option.

- **Panicky feelings**: a few people may experience panicky feelings, often due to a sensation of sinking or feeling they may lose control or are being taken over by the voice. These feelings can often be overcome by doing the exercises more or less upright in a recliner type chair and not closing the eyes.

- **Dislike of one of the voices on the CD**: try another CD; there are many on the market and most cost only a few pounds.

Therapist variables

Yes, that's you! Some people get better results helping people to learn relaxation than others. One of the factors is how they feel about relaxation. If you have never tried it or feel that it is for 'people with problems' or that it's 'not for you' you are unlikely to be able to convince other people to try it. It is important that you have not only tried it but become proficient at using relaxation in difficult situations yourself before you go on to teach it.

It is also important that at each meeting with the person you ask how they are getting on and encourage them to carry on, asking about any improvements they may have noticed in their sleep, their ability to relax, what feelings they get when they do it. Try and spend a few minutes each time emphasising the benefits they can expect. People who are sceptical or ignorant about the benefits of relaxation are less likely to do this.

Breathing

Breathing

Breathing retraining

Why is breathing retraining important? Surely everyone knows how to breathe? If only that were true! We tend not to think of our breathing unless we have problems, but abnormal breathing patterns are fairly common. Before we go any further, it may help to do a simple recap of how we breathe.

Think about what happens during quiet respiration. We know that the lungs are enclosed in a cage made up of the chest wall and the diaphragm. By increasing the cage size, the lungs expand and air is drawn in, and when the cage returns to its resting size air is pushed out. Of the two components involved in increasing the cage size, which is the most important: the diaphragm or the chest wall?

If you answered 'chest wall' you were wrong. The major component of quiet respiration is the diaphragm. The diaphragm at rest is domed, and when it contracts during inspiration it flattens down, increasing the internal size of the cage, which also compresses the abdominal contents, causing the abdominal wall to expand outwards. The chest wall remains still. This relaxed way of breathing is referred to as abdominal (or diaphragmatic) breathing, and is the way babies and children breathe. See Figure 7.1.

Figure 7.1

Diaphragmatic breathing

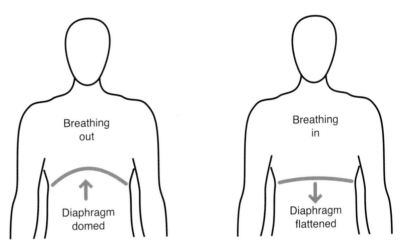

Abdominal breathing depends on the abdominal wall expanding to allow displacement of the gut. If the abdominal muscles are rigid during inspiration, this cannot happen, instead the chest wall must expand more to compensate (Brewis, 1991). We also use the chest wall during inspiration when we need deeper respiratory effort, for example during exercise or when we are excited or upset. In the majority of people there is a mix of abdominal and thoracic breathing depending on what we are doing, but in some people it is thoracic breathing that becomes predominant. Some people go further and develop paradoxical breathing, in which the abdomen moves out during expiration and in during inspiration (and is therefore the reverse of abdominal breathing) (Peper and Tibbetts, 1994). As you can imagine, this is not a very efficient way of breathing and can contribute to feelings of breathlessness.

Chronic disease management for long-term conditions

Other patterns of breathing which are dysfunctional include quick shallow breathing, breath-holding on effort, sighing and gasping, and irregular breathing patterns (Peper and Tibbetts, 1994). These forms of breathing are a part of 'hyperventilation syndrome' (Thomas *et al.*, 2003), which can play a key role in panic (Clark, 1986). So rapid, shallow, upper chest breathing can produce feelings of dizziness, chest tightness, blurred vision and palpitations (Simos, 2002). Yet hyperventilation is incompatible with slow, abdominal breathing (Simos, 2002).

Dyspnoea (significant breathlessness) can affect people with many different long-term conditions, including coronary heart disease and chronic airways disease. In their position statement on dyspnoea, the American Thoracic Society noted that it was not just the severity of dyspnoea that differed between patients, but also the sensation of breathlessness (American Thoracic Society, 1999). Many patients, even when they receive optimal treatment for their underlying problem, continue to experience debilitating amounts of breathlessness (American Thoracic Society, 1999). This observation directs us back to the earlier discussion on disability and impairment; that, again, there is little to link the underlying disease with the degree of breathlessness that patients suffer. In patients who have been taught abdominal breathing, and encouraged to check their breathing often during the day, there has been an improvement in cardiac symptoms and pulmonary function (DeGuire *et al.*, 1996, Gilbert, 2003, Vasiliauskas and Jasiukeviciene, 2004).

Abdominal breathing

Abdominal breathing is a really useful technique for reducing anxiety in any situation. It is worth practising yourself – we all have times when we feel tense! You can easily show the patient how to do this at the first meeting, but the technique needs practice to become automatic.

At first it may be better for the patient to lie down to practise this but it may not be possible to show this at the first appointment. To demonstrate the breathing technique to the patient whilst seated, place one hand on your chest and one on your abdomen. Try to breathe just with the abdomen, just easy breaths, so that as you breathe in your abdomen rises, and as you breathe out your abdomen falls. The hand on your chest should remain still, while the hand on your abdomen should rise and fall with the breathing (see Figure 7.2).

Encourage the patient to check their breathing during the day. The more often that they check and correct their breathing pattern, the more habitual it will become. Some patients find it helpful to set their watch to beep each hour to remind them, at least at first, to check their breathing.

Figure 7.2   ## Abdominal breathing while seated

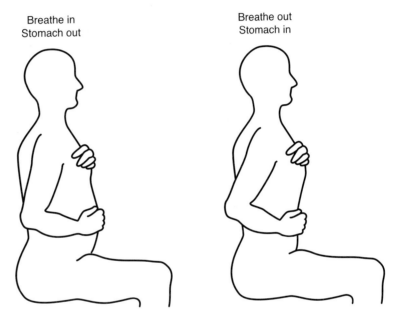

Breathe in
Stomach out

Breathe out
Stomach in

Keep the chest still

Points for reflection

● Consider how you might build in the use of relaxation techniques with the people you support.

● Can you think of anyone you currently support who would benefit from the use of relaxation techniques?

● How might you use breathing retraining in your usual practice?

Chapter 8
Anxiety and depression

Learning outcomes

The chapter aims:

- to assist the reader to recognise symptoms of anxiety and depression in order to facilitate referral back to the general practitioner for further assessment and possible onward referral
- to explore the ways in which anxiety and depression can complicate the management of long-term physical conditions.

Introduction

In this chapter, we first outline the nature of anxiety and depression and discuss how to recognise these conditions. Following this some ways in which anxiety and depression can interact with long-term conditions are described. We then present a case study illustrating CBT work with a depressed patient. Finally some suggestions for further reading and training in CBT are included.

What is depression?

Depression

Depression is characterised by a range of emotional, physical, behavioural and cognitive symptoms. Emotional symptoms include loss of interest and enjoyment, low mood, irritability and feelings of guilt. Physical symptoms include tearfulness or inability to cry, sleep and appetite disturbance, reduced libido and fatigue. Cognitive symptoms include poor concentration and difficulty in making decisions. Behavioural changes include reduced activity and withdrawal. Low self-esteem and reduced self-confidence are also common and a depressed individual may feel hopeless about their situation and the future. Suicidal thoughts commonly occur in depression and there is a risk that such thoughts may be acted upon.

Depression can take a number of forms. It can be classified according to whether it is mild, moderate or severe. The National Institute for Health and Clinical Excellence (NICE) amended guidelines for managing depression; they also identify recurrent and treatment-resistant depression (NICE 2007). In bipolar disorder episodes of depression alternate with episodes of manic behaviour during which individuals experience a sense of euphoric over-confidence alongside impaired judgement which can result in risk taking.

For an account of the experience of depression and an overview of theory and treatment, including CBT, see Wolpert (1999).

Identifying depression

It is important to recognise depression so the person can be referred back to their own doctor for appropriate help. Given that long-term conditions such as diabetes or coronary heart disease increase an individual's vulnerability to depression, it is particularly important to recognise depression in this group of patients. The NICE guideline for depression (NICE, 2007, p. 16) states that 'Screening should be undertaken in primary care or general hospital settings for depression in high-risk groups – for example those with a past history of depression, **significant physical illnesses causing disability**, or other mental health problems, such as dementia' (emphasis added). The guideline (NICE, 2007, p. 16) suggests that a minimum of two key screening questions are asked:

- During the last month, have you often been bothered by feeling down, depressed or hopeless?
- During the last month, have you often been bothered by having little interest or pleasure in doing things?

An affirmative answer to these questions suggests that depression is present. For further information about depression see the NICE guideline for depression (2007), in which Appendix E suggests a series of steps to take in 'Assessing the severity of depression in primary care' and the factors favouring different levels of intervention.

A number of questionnaires are also available to help identify depression. Details of some of these can be found in Chapter 9.

Risk of depression

People with depression are at increased risk for suicide. The NICE guidelines for depression recommend that 'Healthcare professionals should always ask patients with depression directly about suicidal ideas and intent' (NICE, 2007, p. 13). It is important that an affirmative answer is carefully followed up and appropriate action taken, depending on the level of risk. It is important to be aware of local services, for example crisis and home treatment teams. A full discussion of risk management is beyond the scope of this chapter. The reader is referred to the NICE guidelines for depression (2007), the National Suicide Prevention Strategy for England (Department of Health, 2002) and *Safety First* – a report into suicide and homicide by people with mental illness (Department of Health 2001). In line with the recommendations contained within *Safety First (Twelve Points to a Safer Service*, p. 162), all staff should have training in the management of risk (both suicide and violence) every three years.

What is anxiety?

Anxiety

Most of us will experience feelings of anxiety at some time. Some degree of anxiety can be useful, for example, anxiety before an important exam can mobilise us to get down to revision; here anxiety draws our attention to the need to address a problem and make plans to avoid the undesirable consequences of failure. Similarly if a car pulls out in front of us the emergency 'fight or flight' reaction mobilises us to take immediate avoidant action.

A detailed discussion of the diagnostic criteria for the range of anxiety disorders is beyond the scope of this book. NICE guidelines, as they become available, should be consulted. Guidelines have been published for panic disorder and generalised anxiety disorder (NICE, 2004a) and obsessive–compulsive disorder or OCD (NICE, 2005). For a discussion of anxiety disorders, including diagnostic criteria, see Wells (1997).

The experience of anxiety

Some common experiences of anxiety are on a continuum with clinically significant anxiety and can give us some insight into those conditions. For example many people faced with challenging circumstances find themselves worrying about their problems. Although occasional worry is a common and normal phenomenon, for a person with generalised anxiety disorder (GAD) worry and fears about being unable to cope can become pervasive and disabling. Being diagnosed with a long-term condition may understandably provoke various concerns, for example about capacity to work, prognosis and quality of life; however individuals with a propensity to worry excessively may become very anxious and find it difficult to relax. This can sap time and energy, may compromise effective self-management and quality of life and could undermine recovery.

For most of us a persistent physical symptom causes concern, prompting us to seek medical advice. A person with health anxiety or hypochondriasis becomes unduly preoccupied with the meaning of perceived symptoms and repeatedly checks themselves for new symptoms and physical changes. Excessive checking, for example, feeling repeatedly for breast lumps or other anomalies can cause discomfort which may be misinterpreted in alarming ways. The person may compulsively seek reassurance from medical practitioners, family and friends which provides only transient comfort. Others may avoid medically related material, such as might be found in magazines or on TV. Individuals with hypochondriasis are likely to hold erroneous beliefs about health (Warwick and Salkovskis, 1990). An example might be a belief that raised heart rate is dangerous. An individual with such a belief might avoid all strenuous activity and rest excessively, resulting in general unfitness and loss of strength (just like Margaret in Case example 7, in Chapter 3). Health anxiety can therefore complicate effective management of a long-term condition through misperceptions about illness and its management, for example employing avoidance coping behaviours (Holahan *et al., 1995*; James and Wells, 2002). Repeated unnecessary reassurance seeking from health practitioners (Warwick and Salkovskis, 1990) may compromise relationships with medical staff.

Most of us will be familiar with the somatic consequences of anxiety – sweating, rapid heart beat, butterflies in the stomach, etc. In panic disorder such symptoms may be misinterpreted as signalling some immediate physical or psychological catastrophe, triggering thoughts such as 'This is a heart attack' or 'I'm going to lose control'. Often panic attacks are accompanied by hyperventilation (over-breathing) perhaps through attempts to control breathing, e.g. taking deeper breaths. Hyperventilation results in a variety of potentially alarming sensations such as dizziness, tingling sensations and increased breathlessness, which are then misinterpreted in frightening ways. These catastrophic misinterpretations can lead to an escalation of symptoms and a vicious cycle ensues where the person is hypervigilant for signs of physical or mental upset and may begin to avoid situations where they feel vulnerable. Panic disorder can compromise effective management of long-term conditions, for example panic attacks with hyperventilation can provoke or exacerbate asthma attacks (Carr, 1999).

A fear or wariness of dogs, mice or spiders is not uncommon. Others may feel uncomfortable with heights or enclosed spaces. In phobias such fears and the accompanying avoidance can be extreme and may come to dominate a person's life. Phobias can also develop around medical procedures, for example in blood injury phobia, a person may avoid blood tests, injections and other scenarios where blood and/or injury may be encountered. In contrast to most anxiety disorders where blood pressure is elevated, those with blood injury phobia experience a drop in blood pressure when faced with the feared situation and may faint. This has implications for those with a long-term condition, for example complicating routine tests. Ost and Sterner (1987) describe a behavioural method for treating blood injury phobia.

Facing social challenges such as going to a party where we don't know many people or giving a speech or presentation where we feel exposed to the scrutiny of others, may cause anxiety similar to that experienced by a person with social anxiety. In social anxiety people become preoccupied with, and highly self-conscious about, how they are appraised by others. This can lead to avoidance of social situations and increasing isolation. People with long-term conditions may become very self-conscious about changes in their appearance resulting from the problem. Those with, for example, the swollen joints of rheumatoid arthritis, severe skin conditions (e.g. acne or eczema), scars resulting from surgery and the changed facial appearance ('moon-face') associated with use of corticosteroids, may become self-conscious, preoccupied with how they are perceived by others and begin to avoid social situations. Social isolation can increase the risk of depression. The case of Michael (see Chapter 1), an asthma sufferer concerned about using his inhaler in front of others, illustrates the interaction between physical illness and social anxiety.

Finally, many people when leaving the house, maybe to go on holiday, will be drawn back to check – yet again – that the door is locked and the gas switched off. This experience gives a glimpse of what it is like to have obsessive–compulsive disorder (OCD) in which individuals are trapped in a cycle of obsessive, anxiety- provoking thoughts, coupled with compulsive rituals which serve, only temporarily, to reduce anxiety. Intrusive thoughts similar to those experienced by people with OCD are very common but most people do not regard them as significant and dismiss them. In OCD such thoughts are accorded undue significance. Obsessive thoughts typically focus on the possibility of causing harm to self or others and are accompanied by an elevated sense of personal responsibility for avoiding this harm. Compulsions may be observable behaviours, for example excessive washing or cleaning or repeated checking, or they may be covert, as in the silent repetition of a phrase, rhyme or number sequence. For people with a chronic health problem as well as OCD, OCD may be a complicating factor causing exhaustion and elevating stress and anxiety. Self-management could become the focus of obsessions and compulsions, and rituals may encroach on time and energy that would be better spent in effective self-care.

In conclusion, many types of anxiety disorder have been identified; however all individuals suffering from anxiety share concerns about the possibility of immediate or future harm to themselves or others, although the nature of the perceived threat varies considerably from fears of imminent heart attack or similar in panic disorder, to persistent fears that unexplained symptoms might be serious (health anxiety).

Identifying anxiety

The NICE guidelines for anxiety (panic disorder and generalised anxiety disorder, GAD) make the point that 'the constellation of symptoms and signs are nebulous' and that several consultations may be required to define the problem and determine an appropriate course of action (NICE, 2004a, p. 29). GAD may occur alongside other anxiety disorders and depression. Those with panic disorder may restrict their activities and become reluctant to place themselves in situations where escape might be difficult or embarrassing (for example sitting in the middle of a theatre) or where help would be difficult to access in the event of a panic attack. Where such avoidance occurs agoraphobia may also be present. Individuals with panic and other anxiety disorders may also become generally worried or apprehensive and may feel demoralised and depressed because of the restrictive impact of anxiety on their life.

The key criteria for identifying *generalised anxiety disorder* are as follows (NICE, 2004a, p. 29):

- symptoms of anxiety, fear, avoidance and increased arousal
- a six-month period of excessive anxiety and worry plus anxiety symptoms.

The key criteria for diagnosing *panic disorder* are as follows (NICE, 2004a, p. 29):

- symptoms of anxiety, fear, avoidance and increased arousal
- recurrent unexpected panic attacks, plus a month of worry, concern about attacks or a change in behaviour.

A CBT perspective on depression and anxiety

CTB in anxiety and depression

As discussed in Chapter 1, CBT posits a relationship between the way we think (cognition), our emotions and associated physiological reactions and our behaviour. CBT does not suggest that thoughts cause psychological difficulties – a number of factors, such as stressful life events, chronic adversity (e.g. poverty and deprivation), adverse childhood experience (for example bullying or abusive parental behaviour), physical ill health (e.g. chronic pain) and perhaps genetic factors, may all contribute – however beliefs and thoughts can have a powerful role in the development and maintenance of depression and anxiety. A CBT understanding of depression suggests that regardless of the cause of an episode of depression, it is maintained by unhelpful thinking patterns. The thoughts of depressed people typically concern themes of loss and hopelessness. These thoughts centre on the self, the wider world including other people and the future. For example 'I'm letting everyone down', 'I'll never get better', 'I could lose my job', 'My partner will find someone else', 'There's no point', and so on. These thoughts produce and amplify low mood, can result in withdrawal from activity and from other people, and the resulting vicious cycles can intensify and maintain depression. While depressed individuals may be experiencing real adversity and it is essential to understand this, their thinking may nonetheless be distorted – blaming themselves unfairly for their predicament, inappropriately attributing their depression to personal weakness, seeing things in black and white terms, over-generalisation, focusing on the negative, 'catastrophising' (predicting future disaster on the basis of limited evidence) and so on. A CBT approach to depression will typically involve the following elements:

- a thorough assessment including history and assessment of suicide risk
- an explanation of the CBT model of depression
- development of a formulation to help the person make sense of the development and maintenance of depression
- an exploration of the relationship between activity and mood with a view to help the person gradually re-engage in rewarding activities
- identification of the negative patterns of thinking that characterise and maintain depression; thought records may be used to help the person identify and evaluate evidence for and against specific negative thoughts
- behavioural experiments to practically test out new and more balanced perspectives
- a range of other approaches such as problem solving, assertiveness training and sleep management ('sleep hygiene') may also be employed as appropriate
- although CBT for depression is principally a 'here and now' approach, for some individuals further work may be undertaken to address unhelpful core beliefs where these may make the person vulnerable to future episodes of depression
- development of a relapse prevention plan.

More information about CBT for depression may be found in Beck *et al.* (1979), Padesky and Greenberger (1995), and Wright *et al.*

(2006). Greenberger and Padesky (1995), Gilbert, (2000) and Williams, (2001) are self-help guides to managing depression.

Much research has been conducted to understand how anxiety disorders develop and are maintained. The thoughts and beliefs of anxious people are focused on the perceived risk of harm, for example, interpreting a racing heart as meaning there is something physically wrong or attributing undue significance to upsetting intrusive thoughts. These anxious feelings are accompanied by physiological changes (e.g. increased heart rate, muscle tension, sweating, butterflies, shakiness or hyperventilation) which may themselves be misinterpreted and cause anxiety to escalate. For example someone with panic disorder may interpret anxiety symptoms as further evidence that a heart attack or other physical or psychological emergency is imminent, while a person who is socially anxious may think others will notice their unease and judge them adversely. These thoughts, emotions and physical sensations result in unhelpful behaviours. People may seek to avoid or escape anxiety-provoking situations, engaging in a variety of 'safety behaviours' designed to avert feared consequences. While in the short term these may provide some relief, they are ultimately counter-productive as they prevent the person discovering that the feared consequence would not have happened. For example, a person prone to panic attacks may think they are going to faint and therefore sit down, preventing disconfirmation of an erroneous belief. Safety behaviours may actually exacerbate the problem, for example, a socially anxious person may try to plan what they will say rather than listening to others, so conversation becomes stilted and unrewarding, reinforcing their anxiety about how others perceive them. A person with health anxiety may continuously monitor a perceived or actual symptom – this increased attention may amplify the sensations resulting in increased fear.

Avoidance may also mean the person's life becomes severely constricted. For example someone with panic attacks may become housebound, a person with social anxiety may become isolated and someone with a phobia about flying may limit their choices regarding holiday and business travel. Specific cyclical models have been developed for a range of anxiety disorders (see Wells, 1997) and can be very helpful in guiding CBT psychotherapists in their understanding of an individual's difficulties.

A CBT approach to anxiety will typically involve the following elements:

- a thorough assessment including history (it is important to ascertain whether depression is also present and if so to assess this, including suicidal ideation. Where the person has anxiety in combination with depression, NICE (2004, p. 25) advises that '. . . the NICE guideline on management of depression should be followed')

- an explanation of the CBT model of anxiety and provision of information about the problem

- development of a formulation to help the person make sense of the development and maintenance of anxiety

- self-monitoring of anxiety symptoms including triggers, emotional and physical feelings and automatic thoughts; intensity of anxiety may be rated on a scale, e.g. 0–10 where 0 = no anxiety and 10 = extreme anxiety

- the client is helped to identify and challenge unhelpful thoughts

- the concept of avoidance and safety behaviours is introduced

- behavioural experiments tailored to the person's problem will be undertaken to test out new beliefs

- continuing exposure to formerly avoided situations, dropping safety behaviours

- development of a relapse prevention plan.

This is a very general overview of the steps involved in CBT for anxiety. For further information see Beck *et al.* (1985), Padesky and Greenberger (1995), Wells (1997) and Wright *et al.* (2006). Self-help guides to managing anxiety include Greenberger and Padesky (1995), Kennerley (1997) and Williams (2003).

The relationship between chronic ill-health and depression and anxiety

Depression and anxiety in ill health

The relationship of depression to physical illness

There is an established connection between depression and some physical disorders. According to the full depression guidelines (NICE, 2004b, p. 20) '...some physical illnesses do increase the risk of depression, including diabetes, cardiac disease, hyperthyroidism, hypothyroidism, Cushing's syndrome, Addison's disease and hyperprolactinaemic amenorrhoea (Cassano and Fava, 2002).' In addition depression can amplify 'the pain and distress associated with physical diseases, as well as adversely affecting outcomes' (NICE, 2004b, p. 16). NICE, (2004) identifies that death rates for people with myocardial infarction are significantly elevated for those who are depressed following their infarction, both immediately and in the subsequent year (Lesperance and Frasure-Smith, 2000). Death rates are also raised in those with heart failure (Murberg and Furze, 2004). A similarly increased risk of death has been identified when depression occurs in combination with a range of physical illnesses (Cassano and Fava, 2002).

Chronic ill health can impact on an individual's capacity to work, to maintain relationships and engage in leisure pursuits. A person faced with a diagnosis of any potentially disabling or life-threatening condition needs to assimilate this new information. The adjustment process may involve denial, anger, anxiety, depression, despair and eventual acceptance. Moorey (1996) discusses these processes in relation to cancer. He observes that rather than there being an orderly progression through stages, people show considerable variation in the adjustment process. Moorey refers to the work of Horowitz (1986) who

> ...suggests that a major life event challenges our view of the world, and that to come to terms with this we must readjust our internal working models or "schemas" to fit with this new information. The more dramatic the life event... the greater the discrepancy between the new information and existing schemas, and the greater the task of assimilating the new information (Moorey, 1996, p. 455).

The psychological impact of experiencing a heart attack is explored in Bennett (1993) who provides a practical account of the skills required in counselling individuals with heart disease from diagnosis through to the management of risk factors, including stress.

In his discussion of the application of CBT to people experiencing objective adversity, such as a cancer diagnosis, Moorey (1996) argues that there is an important distinction to be made between an individual's natural sadness or upset in the face of loss or ill health, and clinical depression. The principle difference is that depression involves some degree of distorted thinking, for example, undue pessimism. Depression, with reduced activity, de-motivation and a feeling of hopelessness about the future, may directly affect an individual's capacity to take the steps required to manage long-term conditions and requires appropriate treatment. Moorey (1996) describes how CBT approaches may be applied to individuals suffering clinical depression in the face of adversity. This may involve addressing inappropriate guilt and self-blame, managing worry and anxiety and identifying and focusing on areas where the person still has some degree of control and capacity to bring about change.

The relationship of anxiety to physical illness

The NICE guidelines for anxiety (panic disorder and generalised anxiety disorder) note that there is significant co-morbidity between panic disorder and general medical conditions including dizziness, cardiac arrhythmias, hyperthyroidism, asthma, chronic obstructive pulmonary disease, irritable bowel syndrome' (sic, NICE, 2004a, p. 13). Generalised anxiety disorder is also frequently accompanied by 'other conditions associated with stress, such as irritable bowel syndrome' (NICE, 2004a, p. 14).

Anxiety can interact with chronic ill health in various ways. People experiencing chronic pain may find that physical or psycho-logical tension may exacerbate the problem. An unhelpful vicious cycle can then ensue. Broome and Jellicoe (1987) and Cole *et al.* (2005) offer practical self-help guides to living with pain. As discussed earlier, anxious misinterpretations of physical sensations can also complicate management of long-term conditions. For example a person with coronary heart disease who becomes anxious about increases in heart rate when exercising may avoid therapeutic levels of exercise. Such avoidance may compromise recovery (see Margaret, in Case example 7, Chapter 3). For people with asthma, symptoms of anxiety and panic can complicate and exacerbate asthma attacks. Anxiety can also interfere with calm and effective management of symptoms. The example of Michael in Chapter 1 illustrates this. Finally the effects of anxiety and worry can be more indirect. Smokers experiencing anxiety may find it more difficult to quit if they use cigarettes as a coping strategy for managing stress. They may therefore require help to find alternative means of managing anxiety or addressing worries. Food ('comfort eating') may serve a similar function and therefore individuals wishing to lose weight may also benefit from understanding the part that anxiety, worry or stress play in their eating patterns.

Case example 12

Peter

Peter is a 42-year-old man, married to Lisa. They have a son, Simon, who is nine. Peter is a teacher in an inner-city comprehensive school. His wife is a medical secretary. Peter grew up as the youngest of four boys. He would say his parents had a good relationship, on the whole, although from time to time they would row. Peter found this very upsetting, describing their rows as 'open warfare'. He remembers feeling on edge a lot in the family, wondering when the next row would happen. Peter's father was a university lecturer and spent a lot of time at home working hard on various projects and writing his papers and books. Peter felt rather intimidated by his father who was not good at showing affection. Peter felt that his father was mostly interested in his sons' sporting and academic achievements. His mother worked part-time and a series of au-pairs helped care for Peter and his older brothers. His mother was affectionate and loving towards her sons but Peter didn't always feel she had much time for him if he was worried or upset. Sometimes Peter's older brothers would tease him but mostly they got on well. Peter did well academically and was very good at sport, particularly as a sprinter.

Peter had a heart attack six months ago. This had been preceded by a long period of stress at work. Although Peter's initial recovery was good he has not yet returned to work and is becoming increasingly depressed and anxious about his condition and the future. His wife has assumed more and more responsibility for things and is unsure how best to help Peter. She is becoming frustrated because he rarely talks about how things are or how he feels. She is starting to feel resentful because Peter's withdrawal is affecting Simon. Peter has been increasingly avoiding exercise and has not seemed to benefit much from the cardiac rehabilitation programme devised by the hospital.

Peter's family doctor diagnosed depression. Peter was reluctant to take antidepressants. He was referred to Jan, a specialist cardiac rehabilitation nurse who was also a cognitive–behavioural psychotherapist. He tells Jan about his low mood and acknowledges that recently he hasn't felt like doing much including following the cardiac rehabilitation plan agreed on discharge from hospital. Jan asks him to describe a recent time when he felt more depressed.

Peter: It was just yesterday. It was my son's school sports day. I felt really bad around the time we had to go home – and then I felt really stupid about being upset. [*He looks sad.*]

Jan: It sounds like something made you feel really down yesterday and just thinking about it brings back some of the feelings.

Peter: That's right, I'd sort of put it out of my mind until you asked.

Jan: I can see that it's not easy to talk about. In a way the fact that it feels so real again might help us understand what was happening for you but I also want to make sure you feel OK to discuss it...

Peter: Oh yeah, that's fine. It'll probably help to get it off my chest. Anyway, I'd felt OK at first – Simon won a race and I felt really proud of him. He's a really good sprinter – it sort of reminded me of me when I was a kid...

Jan: So at that point you felt OK – proud of your son. What happened next?

Peter: Well it was getting towards the end of the day. I noticed I was starting to feel quite tired. Pretty exhausted actually. And then they announced that it was the Dads' race. Simon asked me if I was going to join in... I told him I wasn't feeling up to it.

Jan: What happened next?

Peter: Nothing much. Simon looked a bit disappointed but he didn't say anything. I suppose he's used to me being boring about things like that.

Jan: When did you notice that you were feeling upset?

Peter: As we were watching the race.

Jan: What was going through your mind?

Peter: I suppose I thought 'I'll never be able to do that again'. [*Looks sad.*]

Jan: And how did that make you feel?

Peter: Sad, upset. I remembered last year when I'd run the race and won and Simon was really excited. I suppose I thought 'I'm letting Simon down'. I was thinking that I'm useless and I'll never get fit again.

Jan: That seems like a pretty upsetting thought. Was there anything else?

Peter: Yeah. I started to feel angry. I was thinking 'Life's not fair'. And then I noticed my heart starting to race. That was scary. I thought, 'Oh no, is this another heart attack?'

Jan: What did you do?

Peter: I told Simon and my wife that we should go home – I made some excuse not to drive... When I got home I went to bed and rested.

Jan: How did you feel then?

Peter: Depressed. I thought things won't get better and I'm letting everyone down.

Jan uses the information that Peter has given to illustrate the vicious cycle of depression and how Peter's harshly self-critical thoughts contributed to his low mood and his withdrawal. This in turn gave rise to further negative thinking (Figure 8.1).

Figure 8.1   **Peter's cycle of depression**

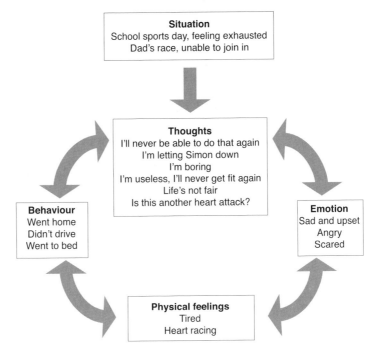

Jan: What do you make of this?

Peter: I can see how it's a vicious circle. But it's true, isn't it? I'm not how I was and I can't do what I used to do with Simon. I'm not getting back to work and recently I haven't felt much like doing any exercise. I am a failure aren't I?

Jan: How do you feel right now when you say these very critical things about yourself?

Peter: Pretty bad. I feel angry and frustrated with myself.

Jan: The thoughts you're having right now seem to be some more examples of how your depression is causing you to be very judgemental of yourself. What I'd like for us to be able to do is to work together to find some ways out of this vicious cycle. Changing one part of the cycle will affect every other part. We might experiment with trying to get a different perspective on the situation. How would you feel about that?

Peter: I can give it a try I suppose.

Jan introduces Peter to the idea of an activity diary. The purpose of the diary is to help Peter discover the relationship between activity and mood. Peter believes that he doesn't do anything useful or enjoyable. There may be some truth in this as reduced activity is a hallmark of low mood. If this is the case a diary can act as a baseline against which the impact of small changes in activity can be measured. Alternatively Peter's low mood may mean he overlooks or cannot recall times when he is more active. A diary can draw attention to the fact that there is some variation across days. Noticing times or activities associated with improved mood can be a starting point for increasing activity likely to give a sense of achievement or enjoyment. Peter decides that he will keep a diary for a week rating his level of depression (on a 0 to 100 scale) against activity. Examples of activity diaries can be found in a range of CBT texts and self-help publications. Jan also gives him some information to read about depression.

At the next session Peter has completed an activity diary. Two illustrative mornings are shown in Figure 8.2.

Figure 8.2   **Peter's activity diary**

Sunday	Monday
7.00 In bed, lying awake, thinking Depression: 80	7.00 In bed awake Depression: 80
8.00 Got up, showered Depression: 70	8.00 Got up. Breakfast with Simon and Lisa Depression: 60
9.00 Had breakfast with Lisa and Simon Depression: 70	9.00 Walked Simon to school Depression: 40
10.00 Helped Simon with school project Depression: 30	10.00 TV Depression: 60
11.00 Watched TV Depression: 50	11.00 TV Depression: 70
12.00 TV Depression: 70	12.00 Washed up breakfast things Depression: 50
1.00 Lunch with Lisa and Simon Depression: 60	1.00 Gardening 20 mins Depression: 30/80
2.00 TV Depression: 70	2.00 TV Depression: 80

Peter brings his activity diary to the next session. He and Jan discuss what can be learned from the diary.

Jan: How did you get on with keeping the diary?
Peter: I managed to remember to do it. It got me down though because I realised how little I'm doing. I feel like a waste of space.
Jan: Keeping the diary has provoked some self-critical thoughts. Perhaps we could look at the thoughts you've been having a little later on. Could we start with taking a look at the diary and seeing what we can learn from it?
Peter: OK. I suppose the thing I noticed was how little I do compared to before the heart attack.
Jan: That is something that can happen in depression. Did you get a chance to read the information about depression and what keeps it going?
Peter: I did. I remember reading that when you're depressed you don't feel like doing much and that leads to the kind of thoughts I've been having about being useless and so on. And then you

feel more depressed and it goes round in a vicious circle.

Jan: That's it exactly. What we need to do is to take a closer look at your diary and see if there's any relationship between how you feel and what you do.

Jan and Peter make the following observations based on Peter's diary.

- Peter tends to feel worse in the morning.
- Peter's mood improves considerably when he is active, doing something he enjoys or considers useful, for example helping his son with homework.

Jan: You were feeling rather better on Monday when you did some gardening but then you rated your depression as 80. What happened there?

Peter: It was a really nice day and I thought I'd get out into the garden and mow the lawn and do a bit of tidying up. It started off OK and I was enjoying myself but I got tired really quickly and had to stop. I remember feeling disgusted with myself. I was comparing myself to how I used to be and I just thought how useless I am now. I went in and watched TV which always makes me feel worse. Even though it takes my mind off things I just think 'what a waste of time'.

Jan: So when you do something that you enjoy or get a sense of achievement from, like the gardening or helping Simon with his project, your mood improves but you get tired and have to stop. That triggers self-critical thoughts and you feel frustrated and depressed.

Peter: That's it.

Jan: What do you think is contributing to your tiredness?

Peter: Well two things. Since the heart attack I tire very easily. And then I read in that booklet you gave me that depression can also lead to tiredness.

Jan: That's right. You mentioned last week that you haven't felt much like doing the exercise programme.

Peter: No, and I feel guilty about that too, like I'm not trying hard enough. And that makes me feel depressed and so I feel even less like doing it.

Jan: So, the diary showed that when you've been more active you've felt better but you get tired and that leads to frustration and low mood. Can you think of anything you might do differently next week that might help you feel better?

Peter: I suppose I could plan to be a bit more active in the week. I really enjoyed spending time with Simon. When we were doing the homework together and when I walked to school with him I felt better about myself.

With Jan's help Peter plans to increase his activity over the next week. They also agree that he will pace himself by building in breaks so that he does not get too tired. He decides to spend some time doing something enjoyable each day with Simon. He also decides that he will go for a short walk each day and will cook the evening meal three nights in the week.

He continues to monitor his activity and discovers that increasing activity is associated with elevated mood. Following this Jan and Peter discuss how Peter can re-introduce his cardiac rehabilitation programme. In addition he noted an improvement in his relationship with Lisa. As Peter's mood and confidence improve he feels ready to contemplate a return to work. A phased return to part-time teaching is negotiated. One year later Peter is teaching three days a week, is enjoying family life and is physically and emotionally well.

Points for reflection

- What are the main symptoms of depression? How would you identify depression among your patients?
- Summarise the ways in which depression might complicate a person's management of a chronic health problem such as diabetes or coronary heart disease.
- How might the different anxiety disorders complicate management of chronic illness?
- How would you identify anxiety among patients on your caseload?

Chapter 9
Assessing needs and outcomes

Learning outcomes

By the end of this chapter you will be able to:

- understand the importance of measuring patient outcomes that reflect their viewpoints
- access different measures to assess outcomes in your patients.

Introduction

As people live longer they are more likely to suffer from a long-term condition, and this has led to an increasing interest in outcomes that are not simply about mortality and morbidity (Fallowfield, 1996; McDowell and Newell, 1996; Wilson and Cleary, 1995). There are aspects of living with a long-term condition that need to be captured in order to have a greater understanding of the effect of the care and information that we, as health workers, provide for people with long-term conditions.

There is also an increasing requirement for health workers to show that they have audited their programmes of care. Audit can help us to identify the strengths and weaknesses of our programmes, showing us where we can improve our performance, and where we can be justifiably proud.

A recent innovation in the audit of the management of long-term conditions is the development of audit datasets for use nationally. For example, there are now available a number of different minimum datasets for use in audit, including those for:

- cardiac rehabilitation
(see http://www.cardiacrehabilitation.org.uk/dataset.htm)

- mental health care
(see http://www.icservices.nhs.uk/mentalhealth/dataset/)
- palliative care
(see http://www.aswcs.nhs.uk/informatics/PalliativeCareMinimum Dataset/)
- smoking cessation
(see http://www.ashscotland.org.uk/ash/4241.html/).

These data are useful for the development of business cases for additions to care, or for highlighting areas of practice that may be improved by changes in methods of delivery of care. If audit data is shared, even anonymously, it enables workers in one area of the country to compare their practice with other similar areas, which may help in obtaining improved outcomes. So audit data can be instrumental in the sharing of best practice.

In this chapter we look at some of the methods that can be used to provide a more complete overview of the effect of promoting self-management in people with long-term conditions.

Quality of life

Quality of life

Improving health-related quality of life is now seen as a worthwhile outcome for healthcare providers (Deyo, 1991; Dunderdale *et al.*, 2005), but is still often not talked about or measured in routine consultations with people with long-term conditions. Do you talk about quality of life in your day-to-day consultations? What do you mean by 'quality of life'?

Clinicians often use measures of functional status (for example, the New York Heart Association Classification or the Health Assessment Questionnaire) and refer to them as 'quality of life' measures, when the two are very different (Roebuck *et al.*, 2001). This represents the biomedical approach to health where health is the absence of disease, not a positive state of well-being.

A generally agreed definition of quality of life is that it is 'a multi-faceted construct that has physiological, psychological, emotional and social components' (Roebuck *et al.*, 2001, p. 766).

Health-related quality of life is concerned with the effects of an illness, including its treatments, as seen from the person's viewpoint (Dunderdale *et al.*, 2005). Health-related quality of life includes aspects relevant to that particular illness experience including reference to vocational status, symptom burden and perception of well-being (Roebuck *et al.*, 2001).

Assessment of health-related quality of life can be undertaken by using a questionnaire. It is useful to measure health-related quality of life as it provides extra knowledge in addition to the more usual clinical outcomes, particularly the way in which the person has viewed their health-related experience (Deyo, 1991).

Point for reflection

There are different reasons why it may be important to measure health-related quality of life. Can you think of two or three reasons?

Reasons why you may wish to measure health-related quality of life:

1. It can be an aid to clinical discussion, as it may open up areas of the patient's life that have been affected by their health which are often not discussed – for example where the person feels that their illness has affected their social lives.

2. As an aspect of clinical audit and service evaluation.

3. As part of clinical research studies, as the importance of quality of life is increasingly recognised.

Quality of life measures are available as either generic or as disease-specific measures. A well-known example of a generic measure would be the Medical Outcomes Trust Short Form 36 questionnaire, better known as the SF-36 (Ware and Sherbourne, 1992). Using generic measures allows for comparison across different illnesses, for example, Rijken and colleagues compared the effect of co-morbid chronic conditions using the SF-36 (Rijken *et al.*, 2005). Disease-specific quality of life questionnaires have greater clinical sensitivity and are more responsive to change in that particular illness (Roebuck *et al.*, 2001). Examples include the European Organisation for Research and Treatment of Cancer (EORTC) questionnaire (Aaronson *et al.*, 1991) and the Minnesota Living with Heart Failure Questionnaire (Rector *et al.*, 1987).

So, how to choose the right questionnaire? One of the easiest ways is to see if there is a recommended minimum dataset for your area of practice that includes a valid and reliable quality of life questionnaire. If it does not, or if there is no minimum dataset in use as yet for your practice, then it is worth looking at reports of quality of life in the patient group that you work with. Is there a review of the different questionnaires available in your area of practice (but be aware that these may be written by people who are developing their own versions, and so open to bias)? What questionnaire is used most often in your area of clinical practice? Do they report that it was valid and reliable in your practice area? Is it easy to use and score?

A good questionnaire for use in clinical practice may differ from one used in research, as there needs to be a balance between how reliably it measures quality of life against how difficult it is to complete and score. If you have difficulty gaining enough detail of a questionnaire (including how to get hold of it) then email or write to the person or team who designed the measure (most journal reports have an address for correspondence) and ask them your questions. Never be shy about doing this, they are likely to be flattered that you are interested in their work. There are very useful books that reproduce and critique questionnaires used in health care, see for example Bowling (2004) or McDowell (2006).

Patient assessment

Assessing beliefs about illness

Patient assessment

One way to assess what people believe about their long-term condition is to ask them open questions, like 'Why do you think that you developed diabetes?' or 'What do you do to manage your daily tasks and activities?'. Asking questions like this means that you will find out about the specific beliefs someone has about living with a long-term condition. This also means that you can give education tailored to those specific beliefs, so that if someone answers in a way that suggests they cope very well, all that may be needed is to praise them on the way they are coping. Conversely, if their answer suggests they are coping in a way that may make their experience worse, then you can help them to deal with that.

However, there are many health workers who do not have the time to undertake a long interview about how someone manages with their condition. For example, practice nurses may be limited to a 10- or 20-minute appointment, during which they must also assess physiological aspects of the condition such as taking a blood pressure, or assessing lung function. It is at these times that using a questionnaire can help to provide a structure to brief interventions to dispel misconceptions. Questionnaires that can be used in such a way include the different versions of the Illness Perceptions Questionnaire (Broadbent *et al.,* 2006; Moss-Morris *et al.,* 2002; Weinman *et al., 1996*); the York Angina Beliefs Questionnaire (Furze *et al.,* 2003) and the more recent York Cardiac Beliefs Questionnaire.

The Illness Perceptions Questionnaire (IPQ): This was based on Leventhal's common sense model of illness behaviour (see Chapter 3), and elicits the illness representations that are included in the model (identity, cause, timeline, consequences and cure-control) (Weinman *et al.,* 1996). The original version was updated in 2002 (the IPQ-R) to address perceived inconsistencies with the first version (Moss-Morris *et al.,* 2002). A further brief version was more recently developed (Broadbent *et al.,* 2006). While the main use of the IPQ has been in research, there have been studies that have used the responses to the IPQ as a starting point for talking about beliefs and dispelling misconceptions (for example, Petrie *et al.* (2002) reported such use in people post myocardial infarction). All of the questionnaires are available from http://www.uib.no/ipq/ as are translations and different disease-specific versions.

The York Angina Beliefs Questionnaire (YABQ): This was developed from patient interviews about angina, and is a questionnaire of specific misconceptions and maladaptive beliefs about living with angina. It is valid and reliable (Furze *et al.,* 2003), and a link was found between people's misconceptions about angina, and their emotional status and physical functioning (Furze *et al.,* 2005). Relatives and friends were also found to have misconceptions about angina (Furze *et al.,* 2002). The YABQ is brief (14 items) and has been successfully used in clinical practice as the starting point for interventions to dispel misconceptions. This questionnaire is reproduced in Appendix 2.

The York Cardiac Beliefs Questionnaire (YCBQ): For those of you working with people with heart disease, or with people who are at high risk of heart disease, this questionnaire has been constructed from common misconceptions of people with angina or after a heart attack, and is taken from patient interviews. The patient can complete this brief questionnaire before you see them, and the questionnaire is then used as a starting point to talk about their beliefs about heart disease. The questionnaire is made up of 22 statements separated into three subscales – generic coronary heart disease beliefs, angina beliefs and myocardial infarction beliefs. The YCBQ is available in two versions, one for use in research and one for clinical practice. Both are reproduced in Appendix 3 with details of their validity and reliability.

Identifying anxiety and depression

Anxiety: As Chapter 8 showed, identifying anxiety is not straight-forward. One of the most widely used measures in clinical practice in the UK for people who have physical illnesses is the Hospital Anxiety and Depression Scale (HADS) (Zigmond and Snaith 1983). This is a simple questionnaire that produces scores for anxiety and depression, with scores below 8 being within a 'normal' range, scores of 8 to 10 being borderline, and scores of 11 and over suggesting 'caseness', that is they are abnormal scores and as such warrant further investigation. The HADS is available from NFER Nelson (www.nfer-nelson.co.uk/) and requires registration with the company and the payment of a fee.

Depression: As Chapter 8 stated, the NICE guidelines include screening questions for depression:

- During the last month have you often been bothered by feeling down, depressed or hopeless?
- During the last month, have you often been bothered by having little interest or pleasure in doing things?

There are also questionnaires to screen for this, including the HADS (see above) and the more recent PHQ9 for the assessment of depression, which is available free of charge from www.phqscreeners.com. The website has directions for how to use this simple questionnaire, which includes versions of the NICE screening questions above.

Goal-setting diary

Earlier, in Chapter 6, we suggested that a goal-setting diary might be useful. We have produced a simple diary template in Appendix 4 just for goal setting; it is not a thought record (see Chapter 1) but it does allow the patient to record their feelings over the week. The diary template is just that – it is up to you to change it or to just take the basic concept and develop one that meets your practice needs. The weekly page could be photocopied for longer-term follow-up.

Using the questionnaires

Clinicians often report that there is too little time to have people complete questionnaires in a consultation or that this will in some way harm the relationship with the person. All the evidence is to the contrary, that people like to fill in questionnaires because it shows that they are receiving the same systematic appraisal as all other people.

It is important to be aware of and sensitive to the possibility that some people may not be able to read, or not be able to read English. This can be got round by accessing the translated version for people who read other languages (many of the more frequently used questionnaires have translations available), or by reading it to people who are unable to read and completing it for them.

There are several solutions to the time problem: questionnaires can be sent to patients before the appointment or they could complete the forms and questionnaires while in a waiting room.

Our evidence is that the time spent ensuring the questionnaire is completed will truly enhance the experience and interaction of the consultation and your interventions in supporting each individual.

Points for reflection

- Consider how you currently assess quality of life of the people you support.
- Could you do anything different based on what you have read in this book?
- How you will audit your practice?

Appendix 1:
Decisional balance sheet

This is useful for discussing the advantages and disadvantages of changing behaviour compared with staying the same (based on Rollnick *et al.*, 1999).

Patient name:

Focus of discussion:

	Decisional Balance Sheet	
	Advantages	Disadvantages
Changing		
Staying the same		

Appendix 2:
The York Angina Beliefs Questionnaire

Overleaf is the York Angina Beliefs Questionnaire (YABQ). This 14-item questionnaire has been found to be valid and reliable among people with stable angina (internal consistency: alpha = 0.81, test–retest reliability: $r = 0.79$) (Furze *et al.*, 2003). Change in angina beliefs over one year was the most significant predictor for physical functioning at follow-up, after controlling for the effects of demographic variables and the outcome variable at baseline, whereas change in frequency of angina did not contribute significantly to this model (Furze *et al.*, 2005). Misconceived and maladaptive beliefs about angina are associated with reductions in both physical and psychological status (Furze *et al.*, 2005).

This questionnaire is not suitable for people who have also had a myocardial infarction. (see the York Cardiac Beliefs Questionnaire in Appendix 3).

Scoring

Items 2, 3, 5, 7, 8, 9, 10, 12 and 13 score as follows:
Strongly agree = 4, agree = 3, don't have any idea about this = 2, disagree = 1, strongly disagree = 0.
Items 1, 4, 6, 11 and 14 are reverse scored, so that:
Strongly agree = 0, agree = 1, don't have any idea about this = 2, disagree = 3, strongly disagree = 4.
The total score range is 0–56, with higher scores meaning more misconceptions. It can be easier to record scores as percentages for ease of comparison; this is done by dividing the raw score by 56 and then multiplying by 100.

Using the questionnaire in practice

The questionnaire takes only a few minutes to complete. For those of you who work in clinics, it is worth sending the questionnaire to the patient and asking them to complete it and bring it with them. Or you can ask them to complete it in the waiting room before you see them. This saves time. Ward-based professionals can give it to the patient and come back later to talk about it. People doing home visits can let the patient fill it in when they get there.

Take the patient through the wrong answers (the correct answers are provided overpage). If someone has a complete set of misconceptions then just talk them through the first few at that meeting. You can target any others at later appointments. Trying to overcome too many misconceptions at once will only confuse the patient.

Make a record of the misconceptions that the patient holds (an example of a misconception tracker sheet for the YABQ is given below). As misconceptions are held by the patient's friends and relatives, it is worth having a relative present so they can then hear the right answers too. It is important to check the patient's misconceptions at every appointment to ensure that the education that you give hasn't been eroded by other people's views.

Appendix 2

The York Angina Beliefs Questionnaire

We want to know your views and beliefs about why people get angina and what they should do about it. It is important that you answer every question. Don't spend too long thinking about your answers – the first thing you thought of is what we want to know.
For each question please tick one box. Please don't leave any out.

	Strongly agree	Agree	Disagree	Strongly disagree	I don't have any idea about this
1. It is not always necessary for people with angina to stop what they are doing when they get angina pain	☐	☐	☐	☐	☐
2. Angina is a kind of small heart attack	☐	☐	☐	☐	☐
3. People develop angina because they have too much stress in their lives	☐	☐	☐	☐	☐
4. There's no need for people with angina to take life easy	☐	☐	☐	☐	☐
5. People with angina should always avoid things that bring it on	☐	☐	☐	☐	☐
6. People with angina should exercise	☐	☐	☐	☐	☐
7. Any sort of excitement is bad for people with angina	☐	☐	☐	☐	☐
8. Angina is caused by a worn out heart	☐	☐	☐	☐	☐
9. If people with angina don't rest when they get angina pain it could be fatal	☐	☐	☐	☐	☐
10. People with angina must stay calm	☐	☐	☐	☐	☐
11. Rest is not the best treatment for angina	☐	☐	☐	☐	☐
12. Too much worry causes people to develop angina	☐	☐	☐	☐	☐
13. Angina pain causes permanent damage to the heart	☐	☐	☐	☐	☐
14. It's usually safe to argue with people who have angina	☐	☐	☐	☐	☐

Explanatory notes for the answers to the YABQ

1. It is not always necessary for people with angina to stop what they are doing when they get angina pain	Some people who experience mild angina prefer to slow down rather than stop completely as this is sufficient to control their angina. If this works then that is fine.
2. Angina is a kind of small heart attack	No, it isn't.
3. People develop angina because they have too much stress in their lives	This is a maladaptive belief rather than a true misconception: people who believe that stress was the major cause of their developing ischaemic heart disease are less likely to alter their risky lifestyles and have greater morbidity than people who acknowledge that their known risk factors need changing. So people who hold this maladaptive belief need help to target their behavioural risk factors. However they also need help to manage their stress as it may also cause them to adopt risky lifestyles (smoking, fatty diets, lack of exercise, etc.).
4. There's no need for people with angina to take life easy	That's right. They should keep up the exercise they do (or increase it slowly if they do none). The main thing is to keep going and build up gradually.
5. People with angina should always avoid things that bring it on	Not necessarily, this could result in the person sitting in the house afraid to do anything. Suggest taking glyceril trinitrate (GTN) beforehand, or breaking the task down into small chunks, doing a little at a time and building up activity levels slowly. It is usually possible to give people combinations of drugs that limit the amount of angina. Recent research also suggests that people who suffer from angina attacks may not suffer as much if they subsequently have a heart attack; the angina may provide a sort of protection.
6. People with angina should exercise	It is very advisable for them to exercise, as people who increase their fitness slowly may reduce the amount of angina that they suffer.
7. Any sort of excitement is bad for people with angina	Believing this could severely limit their quality of life. Giving up fun but exciting things could also contribute to depression.
8. Angina is caused by a worn out heart	It is not.
9. If people with angina don't rest when they get angina pain it could be fatal	Not so. See question 1. However people with angina should be taught how to spot if the pain may be a heart attack and what to do, a great deal of fear is generated because they have not been taught this.
10. People with angina must stay calm	Although this may lead to a more relaxing life it is not strictly necessary. It could affect quality of life and family life if the striving for calm causes bottling up of problems, by either the angina sufferer or their family.
11. Rest is not the best treatment for angina	Rest causes people to become less fit, and this can cause more angina pain, so rest is a poor treatment for angina.
12. Too much worry causes people to develop angina	No, see question 3.
13. Angina pain causes permanent damage to the heart	No, it doesn't.
14. It's usually safe to argue with people who have angina	Believing that it is not safe can cause problems in relationships, and make the family overprotective.

Appendix 2

Tracker sheet for the YABQ

	Initial	1st follow up	2nd follow up	3rd follow up
1. It is not always necessary for people with angina to stop what they are doing when they get angina pain				
2. Angina is a kind of small heart attack				
3. People develop angina because they have too much stress in their lives				
4. There's no need for people with angina to take life easy				
5. People with angina should always avoid things that bring it on				
6. People with angina should exercise				
7. Any sort of excitement is bad for people with angina				
8. Angina is caused by a worn out heart				
9. If people with angina don't rest when they get angina pain it could be fatal				
10. People with angina must stay calm				
11. Rest is not the best treatment for angina				
12. Too much worry causes people to develop angina				
13. Angina pain causes permanent damage to the heart				
14. It's usually safe to argue with people who have angina				

Appendix 3:
The York Cardiac Beliefs Questionnaire (YCBQ)

This is the latest (January 2007) version of the York Cardiac Beliefs Questionnaire (YCBQ). This new misconceptions questionnaire can be used with patients with coronary heart disease and their families and friends. It was developed from patient interviews and is divided into three sections; a section of misconceptions about heart disease, and separate sections on misconceptions about angina and myocardial infarction. The section on heart disease has been shown to have good internal reliability (alpha score of 0.76) and stability ($r = 0.81$). The questionnaire is still under study to find out how predictive it is of ill health.

This 22-item questionnaire comes in two versions, one for use in clinical practice (YCBQ-Clinprac) and one for use in research (YCBQ-Res). *You choose which version of the questionnaire suits your practice.* The questionnaire takes only a few minutes to complete. For those of you who work in clinics, it is worth sending the questionnaire of your choice to the patient and asking them to complete it and bring it with them. Or you can ask them to complete it in the waiting room before you see them. This saves time. Ward-based professionals can give it to the patient and come back later to talk about it. People doing home visits can let the patient fill it in when they get there.

Why are there two versions? Questionnaires for use in clinical practice don't really need sensitive scoring systems. For a beliefs questionnaire all you really need to know is 'Does the patient have this belief and is it right?' In research, we are trying to see if people who hold beliefs more strongly are different to people who don't hold them so strongly, so we need more scoring options. You can decide which version suits you better.

YCBQ-Clinprac

This version is suggested for use in normal clinical practice as it is easier to use. It is scored by ticking either agree or disagree for each question. Overpage is a version of the questionnaire which you can photocopy and use with patients. The form is divided op into sections, so that you can decide how much you want to use. *The first 12 questions should be used for everyone;* they deal with misconceptions about heart disease. The other two sections can be deleted if you prefer (they deal with specific misconceptions about heart attack or about angina). So, if you work in Rapid

Appendix 3

Access Chest Pain clinic you can simply give your patients sections 1 and 3, but delete section 2 (questions about heart attack). If a patient agrees with the statement then that is a misconception EXCEPT for four questions – numbers 6, 7, 15 and 20. For these questions, the misconception is when people disagree with the question statement. These four questions are lightly shaded in grey, and they are in the middle of their scales. With a little practice, you should be able to spot misconceptions at a glance. You don't need to score the scale unless you really wish to for your records. Then, we suggest that you score each wrong idea as 1 and each right idea as 0. The higher the number of misconceptions, the higher the score.

YCBQ-Res

This questionnaire is scored on a Likert scale as follows: strongly disagree = 0, disagree = 1, don't know = 2, agree = 3 and strongly agree = 4. There are four questions that are reverse scored: 6, 7, 15 and 20. These are shaded in grey to make them stand out a little for ease of scoring, and they are sited in the middle of each scale to break up the run of misconceptions (to prevent people just choosing to score the same all the way down the scale). We suggest using all 22 items for research studies, but scoring the scales separately (generic coronary heart disease beliefs – items 1–12, scale score range 0–48; myocardial infarction beliefs – items 13–17, scale score range 0–20; and angina beliefs – items 18–22, scale score range 0–20).

Using the questionnaire in practice

Take the patient through the wrong answers (the correct answers are provided on p 137). If someone has a complete set of misconceptions then just talk them through the first few at that meeting. You can target the other misconceptions at later appointments. Trying to overcome too many at once will only confuse the patient.

Make a record of the misconceptions that the patient holds, (an example of a misconception tracker sheet for the YCBQ is also provided). As misconceptions are held by the patient's friends and relatives, it is worth having a relative present, who can also hear the right answers. It is important to check the patient's misconceptions at every appointment to ensure that the education that you give hasn't been eroded by other people's views.

YCBQ-Clinprac

We want to know your views and beliefs about why people get heart disease (angina and heart attacks) and what they should do about it. It is important that you answer every question. For each question please tick one box. Please don't leave any out.

Section 1: Questions about living with heart disease

	AGREE	DISAGREE
1. People who have heart disease should never get excited or upset	☐	☐
2. People develop heart disease because of worry in their life	☐	☐
3. Rest is the best medicine for heart conditions	☐	☐
4. One of the main causes of heart disease is stress	☐	☐
5. It is dangerous for people who have heart disease to argue	☐	☐
6.. Doing exercise can strengthen the heart muscle	☐	☐
7. Heart disease is often caused by people's lifestyle	☐	☐
8. Heart problems are a sign that you have a worn out heart	☐	☐
9. People with heart disease should take life easy	☐	☐
10. Any sort of excitement could be bad if you have heart disease	☐	☐
11. Your heart is like a battery, the more you do the faster it runs down	☐	☐
12. People who have heart disease should always avoid stress	☐	☐

Section 2: Questions about heart attack

	AGREE	DISAGREE
13. It is dangerous for people who have had a heart attack to exercise	☐	☐
14. People who have had a heart attack must be protected from stress	☐	☐
15. After a heart attack life can sometimes be better than before	☐	☐
16. A heart attack makes a weak area in the heart wall that can easily rupture	☐	☐
17. Once you have had a heart attack you are bound to have another	☐	☐

Section 3: Questions about angina

	AGREE	DISAGREE
18. Angina is a kind of small heart attack	☐	☐
19. Any sort of excitement is bad for people with angina	☐	☐
20. People with angina should live life to the full	☐	☐
21. Every bout of angina causes permanent damage to the heart	☐	☐
22. People with angina should avoid being active	☐	☐

Appendix 3

YCBQ-Res

We want to know your views and beliefs about why people get heart disease (angina and heart attacks) and what they should do about it. It is important that you answer every question. For each question please tick one box. Please don't leave any out.

	Strongly agree	Agree	Don't know	Disagree	Strongly disagree
1. People who have heart disease should never get excited or upset	☐	☐	☐	☐	☐
2. People develop heart disease because of worry in their life	☐	☐	☐	☐	☐
3. Rest is the best medicine for heart conditions	☐	☐	☐	☐	☐
4. One of the main causes of heart disease is stress	☐	☐	☐	☐	☐
5. It is dangerous for people who have heart disease to argue	☐	☐	☐	☐	☐
6. Doing exercise can strengthen the heart muscle	☐	☐	☐	☐	☐
7. Heart disease is often caused by people's lifestyle	☐	☐	☐	☐	☐
8. Heart problems are a sign that you have a worn out heart	☐	☐	☐	☐	☐
9. People with heart disease should take life easy	☐	☐	☐	☐	☐
10. Any sort of excitement could be bad if you have heart disease	☐	☐	☐	☐	☐
11. Your heart is like a battery, the more you do the faster it runs down	☐	☐	☐	☐	☐
12. People who have heart disease should always avoid stress	☐	☐	☐	☐	☐
13. It is dangerous for people who have had a heart attack to exercise	☐	☐	☐	☐	☐
14. People who have had a heart attack must be protected from stress	☐	☐	☐	☐	☐
15. After a heart attack life can sometimes be better than before	☐	☐	☐	☐	☐
16. A heart attack makes a weak area in the heart wall that can easily rupture	☐	☐	☐	☐	☐
17. Once you have had a heart attack you are bound to have another	☐	☐	☐	☐	☐
18. Angina is a kind of small heart attack	☐	☐	☐	☐	☐
19. Any sort of excitement is bad for people with angina	☐	☐	☐	☐	☐
20. People with angina should live life to the full	☐	☐	☐	☐	☐
21. Every bout of angina causes permanent damage to the heart	☐	☐	☐	☐	☐
22. People with angina should avoid being active	☐	☐	☐	☐	☐

Explanatory notes for the answers to the YCBQ

1. People who have heart disease should never get excited or upset	Life with no excitement? Boring! Normal excitement won't hurt them. If they often get angry and upset, they should talk to their cardiac rehab team or practice nurse – they may be able to help.
2. People develop heart disease because of worry in their life	No, worry doesn't cause heart disease – risk factors do. But, if there is worry or stress, something should be done about it. patients can ask for advice from the rehab team or practice nurse.
3. Rest is the best medicine for heart problems	No, rest is not a medicine; too much rest makes the heart unfit, leads to a lack of energy and stamina, and can cause even more problems.
4. One of the main causes of heart disease is stress	Everyday life stress isn't one of the major causes of heart disease. But it can make people miserable and lead to bad habits like smoking and not exercising enough, which do cause heart disease.
5. It is dangerous for people who have heart disease to argue	No, once again most people should aim to live a normal life. Disagreements are part of everyday life. Bottling things up can make them worse.
6. Doing exercise can strengthen the heart muscle	Yes, particularly in the safe way that health professionals can advise about.
7. Heart disease is often caused by people's lifestyle	Yes, an unhealthy lifestyle is the main cause of heart disease.
8. Heart problems are a sign that you have a worn out heart	The heart doesn't wear out. It can be made stronger by being more active.
9. People with heart disease should take life easy	No, patients should live as active a life as possible – it will help to prevent more problems.
10. Any sort of excitement could be bad if you have heart disease	No, normal levels of fun and excitement help to make life worth living.
11. Your heart is like a battery, the more you do, the faster it runs down	No, activity recharges the heart.
12. People who have heart disease should always avoid stress	No, avoiding things that may be fun because of a fear of stress can lead to depression. If help is needed to cope with everyday stress, the cardiac rehab team or practice nurse can help.

13. It is dangerous for people who have had a heart attack to exercise	No, providing that exercise is built up gradually. The cardiac rehab team or practice nurse can advise about this. Being active reduces the risk of more heart problems.
14. People who have had a heart attack must be protected from stress	This can lead to them being excluded from normal social life and work, and may lead to depression. If stress is a problem, then there are ways to reduce its impact.
15. After heart attack life can sometimes be better than before	Yes, particularly if they have attended cardiac rehabilitation, which reduces the chance of early death.
16. A heart attack makes a weak area in the heart wall that can easily rupture	No, the scar tissue which forms after a heart attack is strong and very unlikely to cause any problems.
17. Once you have had one heart attack you are bound to have another one	No, most people who have had one heart attack never have another.
18. Angina is a kind of small heart attack	No, it is very different; angina doesn't leave any damage. The cardiac rehab team or practice nurse can explain the difference.
19. Any sort of excitement is bad for people with angina	Excitement makes life worth living. See the answer to question 1.
20. People with angina should live life to the full	Yes, they may have to accept some limitations but should still get the most out of life that they can.
21. Every bout of angina causes permanent damage to the heart	Stable angina does not damage the heart.
22. People with angina should avoid being active	No, people who keep active reduce their risk of more heart problems.

Tracker sheet for the YCBQ

	Initial	1st follow-up	2nd follow-up	3rd follow-up
1. People who have heart disease should never get excited or upset				
2. People develop heart disease because of worry in their life				
3. Rest is the best medicine for heart problems				
4. One of the main causes of heart disease is stress				
5. It is dangerous for people who have heart disease to argue				
6. Doing exercise can strengthen the heart muscle				
7. Heart disease is often caused by people's lifestyle				
8. Heart problems are a sign that you have a worn out heart				
9. People with heart disease should take life easy				
10. Any sort of excitement could be bad if you have heart disease				
11. Your heart is like a battery, the more you do, the faster it runs down				
12. People who have heart disease should always avoid stress				
13. It is dangerous for people who have had a heart attack to exercise				
14. People who have had a heart attack must be protected from stress				
15. After heart attack life can sometimes be better than before				
16. A heart attack makes a weak area in the heart wall that can easily rupture				
17. Once you have had one heart attack you are bound to have another one				
18. Angina is a kind of small heart attack				
19. Any sort of excitement is bad for people with angina				
20. People with angina should live life to the full				
21. Every bout of angina causes permanent damage to the heart				
22. People with angina should avoid being active				

Appendix 4:
Example of a goal-setting diary

Using your diary

Keeping a diary will help you to keep track of how you are doing with your goals. Below you can write down the long-term goals that you would like to achieve. Once you have set your main goals, set weekly targets that will help you to achieve them. For example: your goal may be that you want to lose a stone before your holiday. Your target could be to lose 1–2 pounds a week.

My main goals are:

1. _____

2. _____

3. _____

4. _____

5. _____

Decide your weekly targets

Break down your main goal into small targets. Make sure that they are attainable and realistic (it is no good targeting to lose a stone in a week – it is not realistic). Do not have too many activities on one day. Targets don't have to be for every day – they can be for once or twice a week, but you need to say which days you are setting them for, for example: to attend a yoga class at 7pm on Thursday.

1	2	3	4	5	6	7	8	9	10
I won't do it									*I'll easily do it*

How likely are you to achieve your weekly targets?

Decide how likely you are to succeed with each target. Using this line, circle the number that matches your confidence in having success with your target; a score of 1 means that you think that you will not succeed with your target, a score of 10 means that you think that you will easily succeed. Only set a target that you are fairly confident you can succeed with (one with a score of 7 or over).

Appendix 4

Fill in the diary every day

Write down how you have done with each target every day on the weekly target sheet. Record what score you gave to your confidence in achieving your target on the target sheet. This lets you see if you have set your targets at the right level. At the end of each week write down how the week has gone on the target sheet. Write down how easy or hard each target was. Are you ready to increase the target? You can write down your thoughts and feelings. Or you can write down questions to ask at your next appointment.

Sample target diary

Please set your targets for the week ahead, and give each target a score for how confident you are that you can achieve this target. Then complete the diary daily to say whether you have achieved your target that day.

Week 1	My target score	Date	Date	Date	Date	Date	Date	Date
1.		☐	☐	☐	☐	☐	☐	☐
2.		☐	☐	☐	☐	☐	☐	☐
3.		☐	☐	☐	☐	☐	☐	☐
4.		☐	☐	☐	☐	☐	☐	☐
5.		☐	☐	☐	☐	☐	☐	☐

How did it go? Did you achieve your targets for each day?

- Was anything too hard?

- Was anything too easy?

- How have you felt this week? (If you have been feeling down or that you couldn't cope, please see your general practitioner or...)

Things I want to ask at my next appointment:

Now please set your targets for next week.

Appendix 5:
Further reading and training in cognitive–behavioural therapy

Numerous textbooks are available which provide an introduction to cognitive–behavioural therapy (CBT) and several of these have been referred to in the text. *Learning Cognitive-Behaviour Therapy: An Illustrated Guide* by Wright *et al.* (2006) comes with a DVD illustrating key CBT skills.

There are also a range of resources available for clients. These include:

- *Mind Over Mood* by Greenberger and Padesky (1995)
- *Overcoming Depression: A Five-Areas Approach,* Williams (2001)
- *Overcoming Anxiety: A Five Areas Approach,* Williams (2003)
- *Overcoming* series published by Constable and Robinson
- Booklets on a range of mental health problems published by Oxford Cognitive Therapy Centre; see http://www.octc.co.uk/information
- *The Mental Health Handbook*, Powell (2000)
- A series of CBT-informed leaflets from the Northumberland Mental Health Trust; see http://www.nnt.nhs.uk/mh/content.asp?PageName=selfhelp

Information about CBT training courses is available from the British Association for Behavioural and Cognitive Psychotherapy (BABCP). See http://babcp.com.

Information about Praxis, a distance learning CD-Rom training package produced for primary care and mental health professionals by Northumberland, Tyne and Wear NHS Trust can be found at http://www.praxiscbt.com.

References

Aaronson, N.K., Ahmedzai, S., Bullinger, M., Crabeels, D., Estape, J., Filiberti, A., Flechtner, H., Frick, U., Harny, C., Kaasa, S., Klee, M., Mastilica, M., Osoba, D., Pfausier, B., Razavi, D., Rofe, P.B.C., Schraub, S., Sullivan, M. and Takeda, F. (1991). 'The EORTC core quality of life questionnaire: interim results of an international field study' in *Effect of Cancer on Quality of Life*, ed. D. Osoba. Boca Raton, Florida: CRC Press, pp. 185–204.

American Thoracic Society (1999). 'Dyspnea: Mechanisms, assessment and management. A consensus statement' in *American Journal of Respiratory and Critical Care Medicine*, 159, 321–40.

Bandura, A. (1994). 'Self-efficacy' in *Encyclopedia of Human Behavior*, Vol. 4, ed. V.S. Ramachaudran. New York: Academic Press, pp. 71–81.

Barlow, J., Wright, C., Sheasby, J., Turner, A. and Hainsworth, J. (2002). 'Self-management approaches for people with chronic conditions: a review' in *Patient Education and Counseling*, 48(2), 177–87.

Beck, A.T. (1976). *Cognitive Therapy and the Emotional Disorders*. New York: Meridian.

Beck, A.T., Emery, G. and Greenberg, R.L. (1985). *Anxiety Disorders and Phobias: A Cognitive Perspective*. New York: Basic Books.

Beck, A.T., Rush, A.J., Shaw, B.F., and Emery, G. (1979). *Cognitive Therapy of Depression*. New York: The Guilford Press.

Beck, C.A., Joseph, L., Belisle, P. and Pilote, L. (2001). 'Predictors of quality of life 6 months and 1 year after acute myocardial infarction' in *American Heart Journal*, 142(2), 271–79.

Bell, J.M. (1998). *Comparison of a multidisciplinary home-based cardiac rehabilitation programme with comprehensive conventional rehabilitation in post myocardial infarction patients*. University of London, PhD thesis.

Bennett, P. (1993). *Counselling for Heart Disease*. Leicester: British Psychological Society.

Bennett-Levy, J., Butler, G., Fennell, M., Hackmann, A., Mueller, M. and Westbrook, D. (2004). *Oxford Guide to Behavioural Experiments in Cognitive Therapy*. Oxford: Oxford University Press.

Bowen, D., Ehret, C., Pedersen, M., Snetselaar, L., Johnson, M., Tinker, L., Hollinger, D., Ilona, L., Bland, K., Sivertsen, D., Ocke, D., Staats, L. and Beedoe, J.W. (2002). 'Results of an adjunct dietary intervention program in the Women's Health Initiative' in *Journal of the American Dietetic Association*, 102, 1631–37.

Bowling, A. (2004). *Measuring Health: A Review of Quality of Life Measurement Scales*. Milton Keynes: Open University Press.

Brewis, R.A.L. (1991). *Lecture Notes on Respiratory Disease*. Oxford: Blackwell Scientific Publications.

Bridle, C., Riemsma, R.P., Pattenden, J., Sowden, A.J., Mather, L., Watt, I.S. and Walker, A. (2005). 'Systematic review of the effectiveness of health behavior interventions based on the transtheoretical model' in *Psychology and Health*, 20(3), 283–301.

Broadbent, E., Petrie, K.J., Main, J. and Weinman, J. (2006). 'The Brief Illness Perception Questionnaire' in *Journal of Psychosomatic Research*, 60(6), 631–37.

Broome, A. and Jellicoe, H. (1987). *Living with Your Pain: A Self-help Guide to*

References

Managing Pain. Leicester: British Psychological Society.

Bundy, C. (2004). 'Changing behaviour: using motivational interviewing techniques' in *Journal of the Royal Society of Medicine*, **97**(Suppl. 44), 43–47.

Burke, B.L., Arkowitz, H. and Menchola, M. (2003). 'The efficacy of motivational interviewing: a meta-analysis of controlled clinical trials' in *Journal of Consulting and Clinical Psychology*, **71**, 843–61.

Butler, A.C. and Beck, J. (2000). 'Cognitive therapy outcomes: a review of meta-analyses' in *Journal of the Norwegian Psychological Association*, **37**, 1–9.

Butler, G. and Hope, T. (2007). *Managing your Mind* (2nd edn). New York: Oxford University Press.

Carr, R.E. (1999). 'Panic disorder and asthma' in *Journal of Asthma*, **36**, 143–52.

Cassano, P. and Fava, M. (2002). 'Depression and public health – An overview' in *Journal of Psychosomatic Research*, **53**, 849–57.

Cigrang, J.A., Severson, H.H. and Peterson, A.L. (2002). 'Pilot evaluation of a population-based health intervention for reducing use of smokeless tobacco' in *Nicotine and Tobacco Research*, **4**, 127–31.

Clark, D.M. (1986). 'A cognitive approach to panic' in *Behaviour Research and Therapy*, **24**, 461–70.

Cole, F., Macdonald, H., Carus, C. and Howden-Leach, H. (2005). *Overcoming Chronic Pain: A Self-help Guide Using Cognitive Behavioural Techniques*. London: Constable and Robinson.

DeGuire, S., Gevirtz, R., Hawkinson, D. and Dixon, K. (1996). 'Breathing retraining: a three-year follow-up study of treatment for hyperventilation syndrome and associated cardiac symptoms' in *Biofeedback and Self Regulation*, **21**, 191–98.

Department of Health (2001). *Safety First: Five Year Report of the National Confidential Inquiry into Suicide and Homicide by People with Mental Illness*. London: Department of Health.

Department of Health (2002). *The National Suicide Prevention Strategy for England*. London: Department of Health.

Deyo, R. (1991). 'The quality of life, research and care' in *Annals of Internal Medicine*, **114**, 695–97.

Diabetes UK (2006). *Diabetes Prevalence 2006*. Diabetes UK.

Doherty, Y. and Roberts, S. (2002). 'Motivational interviewing in diabetes practice' in *Diabetic Medicine*, **19**(Suppl. 3), 1–6.

Drossman, D.A., Whitehead, W.E., Toner, B.B., Diamant, N., Hu, Y.J.B., Bangdiwala, S.I. and Jia, H. (2000). 'What determines severity among patients with painful functional bowel disorders?' in *American Journal of Gastroenterology*, **95**(4), 974–80.

Dunderdale, K., Thompson, D.R., Miles, J.N., Beer, S.F. and Furze, G. (2005). 'Quality-of-life measurement in chronic heart failure: do we take account of the patient perspective?' in *European Journal of Heart Failure*, **7**(4), 572–82.

D'Zurilla, T.J. and Goldfried, M.R. (1971). 'Problem solving and behavior modification' in *Journal of Abnormal Psychology*, **78**, 107–26.

Edwards, J., Mulherin, D., Ryan, S. and Jester, R. (2001). 'The experience of patients with rheumatoid arthritis admitted to hospital' in *Arthritis Care and Research*, **45**(1), 1–7.

Elliot, D.L., Goldberg, L., Duncan, TE., Kuehl, K.S., Moe, E.L., Breger, R.K.R.,

DeFrancesco, C.L., Ernst, D.B. and Stevens, V.J. (2004). 'The PHLAME Firefighters' Study: Feasibility and findings' in *American Journal of Health Behavior*, 28, 13–23.

Emmons, K.M., Hammond, S.K., Fava, J. L., Velicer, W.F., Evans, JL. and Monroe, A.D. (2001). 'A randomized trial to reduce passive smoke exposure in low-income households with young children' in *Pediatrics*, 108, 18–24.

Engel, G.L. (1977). 'The need for a new medical model: a challenge for biomedicine' in *Science*, 196, 129–36.

Ershoff, D.H., Quinn, V.P., Boyd, N.R., Stern, J., Gregory, M. and Wirtschafter, D. (1999). 'The Kaiser Permanente prenatal smoking-cessation trial: when more isn't better, what is enough?' in *American Journal of Preventive Medicine*, 17, 161–8.

Fallowfield, L. (1996). 'Quality of life data' in *Lancet*, 348, 421–2.

Furze, G., Bull, P., Lewin, R. and Thompson, D.R. (2003). 'Development of the York Angina Beliefs Questionnaire' in *Journal of Health Psychology*, 8, 307–16.

Furze, G., Lewin, R., Murberg, T.A., Bull, P. and Thompson, D. (2005). 'Does it matter what patients think? The relationship between changes in patients' beliefs about angina and their psychological and functional status' in *Journal of Psychosomatic Research*, 59, 323–9.

Furze, G., Lewin, R.J.P., Roebuck, A., Bull, P. and Thompson, D.R. (2001). 'Attributions and misconceptions in angina: an exploratory study' in *Journal of Health Psychology*, 6, 501–10.

Furze, G., Roebuck, A., Bull, P., Lewin, R.J.P. and Thompson, D.R. (2002). 'A comparison of the illness beliefs of people with angina and their peers: a questionnaire study' in *BMC Cardiovascular Disorders*, 2(4), http://www.biomedcentral.com/1471-2261/2/4. Last accessed 15.3.08.

Gilbert, C. (2003). 'Clinical applications of breathing regulation' in *Behavior Modification*, 27, 692–709.

Gilbert, P. (2000). *Overcoming Depression*. London: Constable and Robinson.

Gilbert, P. (2006). 'Challenging some myths about CBT' in *BABCP Magazine*, May, 3–5.

Greenberger, D. and Padesky, C.A. (1995). *Mind Over Mood*. New York: Guilford Publications.

Hagan, T. and Donnison, J. (1999). 'Social power: Some implications for the theory and practice of cognitive behaviour therapy' in *Journal of Community and Applied Social Psychology*, 9, 119–35.

Hagger, M.S. and Orbell, S. (2003). 'A meta-analytic review of the Common-Sense Model of Illness Representations' in *Psychology and Health*, 18, 141–84.

Holahan, C.J., Moos, R.H., Holahan, C.K. and Brennan, P.L. (1995). 'Social support, coping, and depressive symptoms in late-middle aged sample of patients reporting cardiac illness' in *Health Psychology*, 14(2), 152–63.

Horowitz, M.J. (1986). *Stress Response Syndromes*. Northvale, NJ: Aronson.

James, A. and Wells, A. (2002). 'Death beliefs, superstitious beliefs and health anxiety' in *British Journal of Clinical Psychology*, 41, 43–53.

Jones, P., Quirk, F.H., Baveystock, C.M. and Littlejohns, P. (1992). 'A self-complete measure of health status for chronic airflow limitation – the St. George's Respiratory Questionnaire' in *American Review of Respiratory Disease*, 145, 1321–27.

Kennerley, H. (1997). *Overcoming Anxiety*. London: Constable and Robinson.

Kennerley, H. (2007). *Socratic Method*. Oxford: Oxford Cognitive Therapy Centre.

References

Lane, D., Carroll, D., Ring, C., Beevers, D.G. and Lip, G.Y.H. (2000). 'Do depression and anxiety predict recurrent coronary events 12 months after myocardial infarction?' in *Quarterly Journal of Medicine*, 93, 739–44.

Lesperance, F. and Frasure-Smith, N. (2000). 'Depression in patients with cardiac disease: a practical review' in *Journal of Psychosomatic Research*, 48, 379–91.

Leventhal, H. and Cameron, L. (1987). 'Behavioral theories and the problem of compliance' in *Patient Education and Counseling*, 10, 117–38.

Leventhal, H., Benyamini, Y., Brownlee, S., Diefenbach, M., Leventhal, E.A., Patrick-Miller, L. and Robitaille, C. (1997). 'Illness representations: theoretical foundations' in *Perceptions of Health and Illness*, ed. K.J. Petrie and J.A. Weinman. Amsterdam, The Netherlands: Harwood Academic Publishers, pp. 19–45.

Leventhal, H., Diefenbach, M. and Leventhal, EA. (1992). 'Illness cognition: using common sense to understand treatment adherence and affect cognition interactions' in *Cognitive Therapy and Research*, 16, 143–63.

Leventhal, H., Meyer, D. and Nerenz, D. (1980). 'The common sense representation of illness danger' in *Contributions to Medical Psychology*, Vol. 2, ed. S. Rachman. New York: Pergamon Press, pp. 17–30.

Lewin, B. (1997). 'The psychological and behavioural management of angina' in *Journal of Psychosomatic Research*, 43(5), 453–62.

Lewin, B., Cay, E.L., Todd, I., Soryal, I., Goodfield, N., Bloomfield, P. and Elton, R. (1995). 'The Angina Management Programme: a rehabilitation treatment' in *British Journal of Cardiology*, September, 221–6.

Lewin, B., Robertson, I.H., Cay, E.L., Irving, J.B. and Campbell, M. (1992). 'Effects of self-help post-myocardial-infarction rehabilitation on psychological adjustment and use of health services' in *Lancet*, 339, 1036–40.

Lewin, R.J.P., Furze, G., Robinson, J., Griffith, K., Wiseman, S., Pye, M. and Boyle, R. (2002). 'A randomised controlled trial of a self-management plan for patients with newly diagnosed angina' in *British Journal of General Practice*, 52, 194–201.

Linton, S.J. and Boersma, K. (2004). 'The role of fear-avoidance in the early identification of patients risking the development of disability' in *Understanding and Treating Fear of Pain*, ed. G.J.G. Asmundson, J.W. Vlaeyen and G. Crombez. Oxford: Oxford University Press.

Locke, E.A. and Latham, G.P. (2002). 'Building a practically useful theory of goal setting and task motivation' in *American Psychologist*, 57, 705–717.

Maeland, J.G. and Havik, O.E. (1989). 'After the myocardial infarction. A medical and psychological study with special emphasis on perceived illness' in *Scandinavian Journal of Rehabilitation Medicine* 22(Suppl.), 1–87.

McCambridge, J. (2004). 'Motivational interviewing is equivalent to more intensive treatment, superior to placebo, and will be tested more widely' in *Evidence Based Mental Health*, 7(2), 52.

McCormick, A., Fleming, D. and Charlton, J. (1995). *Morbidity Statistics from General Practice. 4th National Study 1991–1992*. London: HMSO.

McDowell, I. (2006). *Measuring Health: A Guide to Rating Scales and Questionnaires*, 3rd edn. Oxford: Oxford University Press.

McDowell, I. and Newell, C. (1996). *Measuring Health: A Guide to Rating Scales and Questionnaires*. Oxford: Oxford University Press.

Mearns, D. and Thorne, B. (1992). *Person-Centred Counselling in Action*. London: Sage Publications.

Miller, W.R. and Rollnick, S. (2002). *Motivational Interviewing: Preparing People for Change*. New York: The Guilford Press.

Moorey, S. (1996). 'When bad things happen to rational people: Cognitive therapy in adverse life circumstances' in *Frontiers of Cognitive Therapy*, ed. P. Salkovskis. New York: Guilford Press, pp. 450–69.

Moss-Morris, R., Weinman, J., Petrie, K. J., Horne, R., Cameron, L.D. and Buick, D. (2002). 'The revised Illness Perception Questionnaire (IPQ-R)' in *Psychology and Health*, 17, 1–16.

Murberg, T.A. and Furze, G. (2004). 'Depressive symptoms and mortality in patients with congestive heart failure: A six-year follow-up study' in *Medical Science Monitor*, 10(12), CR643–8.

NICE (2004a). *Clinical Guideline 22 – Anxiety: Management of anxiety (panic disorder, with or without agoraphobia, and generalised anxiety disorder) in adults in primary, secondary and community care*. London: National Institute for Health and Clinical Excellence.

NICE (2004b). *Clinical Guideline 23 – Depression: Management of depression in primary and secondary care*. London: National Institute for Health and Clinical Excellence.

NICE (2005). *Clinical Guideline 31 – Obsessive–compulsive disorder: core interventions in the treatment of obsessive–compulsive disorder and body dysmorphic disorder*. London: National Institute for Health and Clinical Excellence.

NICE (2007). *Clinical Guideline 23 (amended) – Depression: Management of depression in primary and secondary care*. London: National Institute for Health and Clinical Excellence.

Ost, L.G. and Sterner, U. (1987). 'Applied tension: A specific behavioral method for treatment of blood phobia' in *Behaviour Research and Therapy*, 25, 25–9.

Padesky, C.A. (1993). 'Socratic questioning: changing minds or guiding discovery?' *European Congress of Behavioural and Cognitive Therapies*: Keynote address, London, 24 September, available at: http://www.padesky.com/clinical corner/pubs.htm#Socratic%20Questioning. Last accessed 15.3.08.

Padesky, C. A. and Greenberger, D. (1995). *Clinicians Guide to Mind Over Mood*. New York: Guilford Publications.

Padesky, C.A. and Mooney, K.A. (1990). 'Clinical tip: Presenting the cognitive model to clients' in *International Cognitive Therapy Newsletter*, 6, 13–14.

Peper, E. and Tibbetts, V. (1994). 'Effortless diaphragmatic breathing' in *Physical Therapy Products*, 6(2), 67–71, available at: http://www.aapb.org/files/public/PeperTibbetseffortlessdiaphragmatic.pdf. Last accessed 15.3.08.

Persons, J.B. (1989). *Cognitive Therapy in Practice: A Case Formulation Approach*. New York: Norton.

Petersen, S., Peto, V., Scarborough, P. and Rayner, M. (2005). *Coronary Heart Disease Statistics*. London: British Heart Foundation.

Petrie, K.J., Cameron, L.D., Ellis, C.J., Buick, D. and Weinman, J. (2002). 'Changing illness perceptions after myocardial infarction: An early intervention randomized controlled trial' in *Psychosomatic Medicine*, 64, 580–6.

Petrie, K.J., Weinman, J., Sharpe, N. and Buckley, J. (1996). 'Role of patients' view of their illness in predicting return to work and functioning after myocardial infarction: a longitudinal study' in *BMJ*, 312, 1191–4.

Powell, T. (2000). *The Mental Health Handbook*. Bicester: Speechmark Publishing Ltd.

References

Prochaska, J.O. and DiClemente, C.C. (1983). 'Stages and processes of self-change of smoking: toward an integrative model' in *Journal of Consulting and Clinical Psychology*, 51, 390–5.

Prochaska, J.O. and DiClemente, C.C. (1984). *The Transtheoretical Approach: Crossing Traditional Boundaries of Change*, Homewood, Illinois: Dow Jones-Irwin.

Prochaska, J.O., Diclemente, C.C. and Norcross, J.C. (1992). 'In search of how people change: applications to addictive behaviours' in *American Psychologist*, 47, 1102–14.

Ready, A.E., Eynon, R.B. and Cunningham, D.A. (1981). 'Effect of interval training and detraining on anaerobic fitness in women' in *Canadian Journal of Applied Sports Science*, 6, 114–18.

Rector, T.S., Kubo, S.H. and Cohn, J.N. (1987). 'Patients self-assessment of their congestive heart failure: content, reliability and validity of a new measure – The Minnesota Living with Heart Failure questionnaire' in *Heart Failure*, 3, 198–209.

Resnicow, K., Jackson, A., Wang, T., De, A.K., McCarty, G., Dudley, W.N. and Baranowski, T. (2002). 'A motivational interviewing intervention to increase fruit and vegetable intake through Black churches: results of the Eat for Life trial' in *American Journal of Public Health*, 91, 1686–93.

Rijken, M., van Kerkhof, M., Dekker, J. and Schellevis, F.G. (2005). 'Comorbidity of chronic diseases' in *Quality of Life Research*, 14, 45–55.

Roebuck, A., Furze, G. and Thompson, D.R. (2001). 'Health-related quality of life after myocardial infarction: an interview study' in *Journal of Advanced Nursing*, 34, 787–94.

Rollnick, S., Butler, C.C. and Stott, N. (1997). 'Helping smokers make decisions: the enhancement of brief intervention for general medical practice' in *Patient Education and Counseling*, 31, 191–203.

Rollnick, S., Mason, P. and Butler, C. (1999). *Health Behaviour Change: A Guide for Practitioners*. London: Churchill Livingstone.

Safran, J. and Segal, Z. (1996). *Interpersonal Process in Cognitive Therapy*. Northvale, New Jersey: Aronson.

Shinitzky, H.E. and Kub, J. (2001). 'The art of motivating behaviour change: the use of motivational interviewing to promote health' in *Public Health Nursing*, 18, 178–85.

Simos, G. (2002). 'Cognitive behaviour therapy for panic disorder' in *Cognitive Behaviour Therapy: A Guide for the Practising Clinician*, ed. G. Simos. Hove: Brunner-Routledge.

Smith, S.S., Jorenby, E.D., Fiore, MC., Anderson, J.E., Mielke, M.M., Beach, K.E., Piasecki, T.M. and Baker, T.B. (2001). 'Strike while the iron is hot: can stepped-care treatments resurrect relapsing smokers?' in *Journal of Consulting and Clinical Psychology*, 69, 429–39.

Smith, T., Follick, M. and Korr, K. (1984). 'Anger, neuroticism, type A behaviour and the experience of angina' in *British Journal of Medical Psychology*, 57, 249–52.

Stang, P., Lydick, E., Silberman, C., Kempel, A. and Keating, E. (2000). 'The prevalence of COPD using smoking rates to estimate disease frequency in the general population' in *Chest*, 117, 354S–59S.

Stotts, A.L., Diclemente, C.C. and Dolan-Mullen, P. (2002). 'One-to-one: a motivational intervention for resistant pregnant smokers' in *Addictive Behaviors*, 27, 275–92.

Thomas, M., McKinley, R.K., Freeman, E., Foy, C., Prodger, P. and Price, D. (2003). 'Breathing retraining for dysfunctional breathing in asthma: a randomised controlled trial' in *Thorax*, **58**(2), 110–15.

Tomkins, S. and Collins, A. (2006). *Promoting Optimal Self-care*. Dorset: Dorset and Somerset Strategic Health Authority.

Vasiliauskas, D. and Jasiukeviciene, L. (2004). 'Impact of a correct breathing stereotype on pulmonary minute ventilation, blood gases and acid–base balance in post-myocardial infarction patients' in *European Journal of Cardiovascular Prevention and Rehabilitation*, **11**, 223–7.

Villani, G.Q., Capucci, A. and Piepoli, M.F. (2000). 'Emerging concepts in exercise training in chronic heart failure' in *Italian Heart Journal*, **1**, 795–800.

Vlaeyen, J.W.S. and Linton, S.J. (2000). 'Fear-avoidance and its consequences in chronic musculoskeletal pain: A state of the art' in *Pain*, **85**, 317–32.

von Bertanlaffy, L. (1975). *Perspectives on General System Theory*. New York, NY: George Braziller, Inc.

Waddington, L. (2002). 'The therapy relationship in cognitive therapy: a review' in *Behavioural and Cognitive Psychotherapy*, **30**, 179–91.

Wakefield, M., Oliver, I. and Rosenfeld, E. (2004). 'Motivational interviewing as a smoking cessation intervention for patients with cancer: a randomized controlled trial' in *Nursing Research*, **53**, 396–405.

Ware, J.E. and Sherbourne, C.D. (1992). 'The MOS 36-item Short Form Health Survey (SF-36): Conceptual framework and item selection' in *Medical Care*, **30**, 473–83.

Warwick, H.M.C. and Salkovskis, P.M. (1990). 'Hypochondriasis' in *Behaviour Research and Therapy*, **28**, 105–17.

Weinman, J., Petrie, K.J., Moss-Morris, R. and Horne, R. (1996). 'The Illness Perception Questionnaire: a new method for assessing the cognitive representation of illness' in *Psychology and Health*, **11**, 431–45.

Wells, A. (1997). *Cognitive Therapy of Anxiety Disorders*. Chichester: John Wiley and Sons.

Whitehead, D. (2001). 'Health education, behavioural change and social psychology: nursing's contribution to health promotion?' in *Journal of Advanced Nursing*, **34**(6), 822–32.

Williams, C. (1997). 'A cognitive model of dysfunctional illness behaviour' in *British Journal of Health Psychology*, **2**, 153–65.

Williams, C.J. (2001). *Overcoming Depression: A Five Areas Approach*. London: Hodder Arnold.

Williams, C.J. (2003). *Overcoming Anxiety: A Five Areas Approach*. London: Hodder Arnold.

Wilson, I. and Cleary, P. (1995). 'Linking clinical variables with health-related quality of life' in *Journal of the American Medical Association*, **273**, 59–65.

Wolpert, L. (1999). *Malignant Sadness: The Anatomy of Depression*. London: Faber and Faber.

Wood, P. (1980). *International Classification of Impairments, Disabilities and Handicaps*. Geneva: World Health Organization.

Wright, JH., Basco, M. and Thase, M.E. (2006). *Learning Cognitive–Behavior Therapy: An Illustrated Guide*. Arlington, VA: American Psychiatric Publishing Inc.

Wynn, A. (1967). 'Unwarranted emotional distress in men with ischaemic heart disease' in *Medical Journal of Australia*, **2**, 847–51.

Zigmond, A.S. and Snaith, R.P. (1983). 'The Hospital Anxiety and Depression Scale' in *Acta Psychiatrica Scandinavica*, **67**, 361–70.

Index

Index

Index